On Being Born
and Other Difficulties

On Being Born

and Other Difficulties

F. GONZÁLEZ-CRUSSI

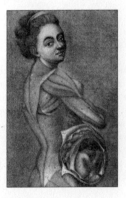

THE OVERLOOK PRESS

Woodstock & New York

First published in the United States in 2004 by
The Overlook Press, Peter Mayer Publishers, Inc.
Woodstock & New York

WOODSTOCK:
One Overlook Drive
Woodstock, NY 12498
www.overlookpress.com
[for individual orders, bulk and special sales, contact our Woodstock office]

NEW YORK:
141 Wooster Street
New York, NY 10012

∞ The paper used in this book meets the requirements for paper
permanence as described in the ANSI Z39.48-1992 standard.

Library of Congress Cataloging-in-Publication Data

Gonzalez-Crussi, F.
On being born and other difficulties / F. Gonzalez-Crussi.
p. cm.
Includes bibliographical references
1. Birth (Philosophy) I. Title.
BD443.G66 2004   618.4—dc22   2004043424
Book design and type formatting by Bernard Schleifer
Printed in the United States of America
ISBN 1-58567-449-4

Contents

ACKNOWLEDGMENT

The author insists in expressing his profound gratitude to the John Simon Guggenheim Memorial Foundation for its generous help. The Fellowship support he received from September 2000 to February 2001 was more than purely material assistance: it constituted a stimulus for undertaking studies that otherwise would not have been possible, and which sparked ideas that will continue to bear fruit beyond the scope of this work.

To Begin at the Beginning . . .
or Almost

WHERE DO WE COME FROM? THE QUESTION ARISES, sooner or later, in every growing child. However, the terms of the enquiry were not always posed in quite the same way. Today, this query leads by natural extension into asking how life started in the world. But this was not always so: in remote times the puzzle would not have taken shape so readily in the mind, for the entire frame of reference was different.

At present, life is viewed as a wondrously subtle process: the result of influences so complex, and phenomena so delicately coordinated, as to boggle the imagination. That this stupendous equilibrium should have arisen in an inanimate universe seems inconceivable. Life is a "miracle," as the trite saying goes. But long, long ago, life was taken for granted, and to enquire about its origin must have struck the human mind as absurd, a ridiculous, useless investigation. What was obviously a problem was to account for death. *This* was the real enigma. That life might cease to exist: this, and only this, seemed to clamor for a rational explanation.

Indeed, the universe seems very much alive. Everywhere we look, we confront manifestations that we feel compelled to call vital. The wind seems alive: its moods change, now streaming forth gently in a soft breeze, now howling frighteningly through blasted, bare and cleft rocks. The clouds seem alive: they roll, they scatter, and stay up or rain down over things manifold. The rivers are alive, since they are animated with perpetual movement, a show of life as evident as that of the trees on its banks, which wave their boughs, and lose their foliage and regrow it. All things in nature emit sounds, or are subject to unceasing rounds of change. Even the stones, that we take to symbolize all that is lifeless and inert, our forbears must have thought infused with life, seeing that they may look as gloomy as specters in the evening, and emblazoned with gold in the noonday, or wrapped in crimson cloaks at dusk. Beneath them, or inside them, one may discover all manner of crawling insects and other creatures. It was natural to assume that the rocks had engendered these beings. And if the rocks could engender, the rocks were alive: they were one more living entity in the nearly infinite catalogue of living things of the universe.

If the universe is alive, and life is "a given," how could death be? Life being omnipresent, eternal, ever flowing, death was inconceivable: it was a monstrous anomaly. A veritable scandal. Nonetheless, it existed. Alas, who would deny it? Its inexorable reminder was there all the time. It was in order to soothe the pain produced by this distressing reality that men turned to religion. This is why all early religions professed belief in some kind of immortality. And the remedy worked well, for so long as mankind was ruled by a predominantly religious outlook. But, in the West, the religious turn of the collective mind changed, as is well known, in the Renaissance. Thenceforward never did we look at Nature in quite the same way. Whereas before the explanations of myth or religion had sufficed, from then on people insisted on concrete ideas conformable to the data supplied by the senses.

Compare, by way of illustration of the change, two paintings, one medieval, and one from the Renaissance. Take, for instance, a Virgin Mary by Giotto such as she appears in the frescoes of Padua's Arena Chapel, highly idealized, nimbed in resplendent glory and wrapped in abstract drapery. Look then at one of the naked Venuses of Renaissance painters, say the *Venus of Urbino* by Titian: fleshy, voluptuous and Circean to distraction. Is there any doubt that the new mentality had renounced symbolization in favor of representation?

Nor was this change impacting the Western world only. In the Renaissance, the first missionaries who arrived in China to propagate the Christian faith brought with them paintings of religious subjects. Huge crowds thronged the churches, and the priests were persuaded that the "heathens" had been swayed by the power of the true religion. They were soon disappointed. The natives had come to see the "foreign pictures;" for they had never seen anything remotely like those easels. Not that they were masterpieces: most were the handiwork of mediocre amateurs, in many cases the missionaries themselves. But Westerners had discovered the laws of perspective, the use of tonal values, *chiaroscuro*, and compositional strategies that achieved arresting results. Reality was represented with striking vigor, in a way that had no precedent in the whole pictorial tradition of the Orient. What occurred in art also happened in other areas of human endeavor. The "objective" turn of mind had arrived.

In science this meant, among other things, that life would no longer be considered "a given." It had to be explained. Life came to be thought of as having emerged from primitive constituents that were themselves lifeless. This view was the opposite of that which existed in more primitive, and more blissful times. The universe therefore changed from mostly living to mostly dead.

Romantic spirits, such as Frederick von Schlegel (1772-1829), were bound to dislike the new stance. He suggested that the human mind is afflicted with this "peculiar error," that it carries the idea of death deeply ingrained in its texture, and transfers it to everything with which it comes in contact. In effect, it seems a sad affair to demote life from all-encompassing, eternal force, to secondary phenomenon. The modern scientific scheme views it as neither very old nor necessarily enduring, since it often appears to be on the verge of extinction. For even if one grants that the fossilized procaryotic bacteria found in the Transvaal prove that life already existed on earth three and one-half billion years ago, this would still be a short duration by reference to the grandiose scale of geologic time and the history of the universe. And whereas the finding of bacteria living in springs of boiling water or the darkest regions of the ocean floor provokes wonderment, it must be owned that life occupies only a thin crust of our planet, not most of its bulk, and that our planet is but a speck in the cold, seemingly lifeless vastness of sidereal space. We thus find ourselves forlorn in a Nature that, as Schlegel[1] put it, is but "a colossal mountain range of petrified mummies," and strain ourselves to explain how life could have originated from this "pyramid of graves."

How, indeed, was life possible? This is one of the greatest questions for biology, perhaps *the* greatest of all enigmas, and the modern counterpart to the former bewilderment upon the origin of death. In the contemporary scientific view, life came about by assembly of lifeless constituents. Presumably, the earth was at one time a very desolate place: a hallucinating, storm-tossed waste, the Apocalyptic landscape for the explosions of thunder and the fiery roar of volcanoes. The continents shifted, and the ensuing tumultuous upheavals saw the raising of blossomless crags that no creature ever trod, and enormous cliffs rifled by the dark eons of prehistory. Naught but the flames of the sun and a torrential rain fell hither. And this barren, forbidding place was enveloped in an atmosphere without oxygen, but containing ammonia, carbon dioxide, methane, and hydrogen. Since there was no ozone layer, nothing screened the ultraviolet radiation of the sun. Hence the molecules that existed in this air were kept in a state of precarious equilibrium. Add to this the occurrence of high-energy jolts, as in the electric discharges of lightning, and you have the conditions necessary to foster the synthesis of organic molecules.

Aleksandr Oparin (1894-1980), Russian savant and leader in the investigation of the origin of life, emphasized that sound hypotheses in this field should be built upon experiments conducted in conditions that reproduce, as closely as possible, the conditions thought to exist on earth before the appearance of living beings. It goes without saying that no investigator could have at his disposal a world without living creatures, immersed in toxic gases, and still shaken by the cataclysms and telluric revolutions of its earliest age. Otto Warburg (1883-1970), Nobel prize winner for his research in physiology (1931), tackled the problem by devising a chamber that reproduced the conditions thought to have existed on the primitive earth. Vaporized water and a mixture of the critical gases simulating the primitive atmosphere were introduced in the chamber, and electric discharges were passed through. Molecules formed as a result of this procedure, that are known building blocks of living beings.

Of Warburg the story is told that he kept the sealed glass chambers for his experiments on his shelves, and when asked what these contrivances were for, he answered—I wish to believe not in jest—that they were for the study of spontaneous generation.[2] He was not lying. For if we ask, as children do, where do we come from, and we are told that we come from our parents, our minds automatically slide on a long retrospective slope: our parents came from our grandparents, who came from our great-grandparents, who themselves were born to our great-great-grandparents, and so on. Yet, this is not an infinite regression: there must come a time when we can retreat no farther. If we go back billions of years in evolutionary history—and our imagination has this admirable faculty, that it can make us swim upstream in the river of time, like preternatural spawning salmons, for however long we fancy—we shall come to the time when no living forms at all are to be seen anywhere. That is to say, we must inevitably come to the time when life began in a dead universe. Thus, life emerged somehow from non-living matter, just as the proponents of spontaneous generation argued when they held that grubs formed from decomposing carrion, and worms from muddy earth.

The original substratum was what scientists are in the habit of graphically calling "the primeval soup." And an unappetizing soup it may have been, composed of the prehistoric oceans with the dissolved mixture of primitive chemicals from which larger organic molecules evolved. Here, once Carbon atoms came into being (by modification of Helium, we are told), a whole array of possibilities lay open. For Carbon atoms, as students of organic chemistry soon learn—by painful experience, some might add—link with each other via their quadruple bonds to make up an astounding number of structures. They can attach to each other linearly, in lengthy chains, or less monotonously, in multi-branched strings. They may form long lines that fold back upon themselves as rings and polyhedrons. Or they may assemble in more inventive combinations, giving rise to compounds that look like boats, chairs, and even elegant geodesic domes with multiple hexagonal faces, as in *Buckminsterfullerene*, the so-called "Bucky balls." It could not have been long before Carbon atoms joined each other in symmetrical molecules that could be split into two equal halves.

The day these molecules incorporated mechanisms that foster this reiterative halving and rejoining, is perhaps the first adumbration of reproduction, since thereby the generation was ensured of new entities made in the semblance of the parent source. And the time when this chemical process could proceed of its own momentum, is perhaps the time when we can begin to speak of "life," in a certain sense. I mean the sense conferred to it by the Cartesian philosophers. Thus,

Malebranche (1638-1715) declared that "the life of bodies, of whatever kind these may be, can consist only in the movement of their parts . . ." For to Cartesians it is of no consequence how subtle or abstruse are the substances that account for the complex physiology of an animal; still, "this matter can be no more perfect than that which activates the springs of a watch or that which causes the weights in the mechanism of a horologe, which is the principle of their life, or to speak like everyone, of their movement."[3]

Did life really come about in this way? Were the original living forms self-replicating complex molecules, perhaps comparable to what we now call "prions" and "viruses"? It must be owned that when it comes to ascertaining facts sundered from us by the chasm of years beyond all common experience, and enshrouded in almost unimaginable antiquity, a dash of healthy skepticism will not seem unbecoming. Be that as it may, the primitive life-forms evolved the means to fence in their inner self and fence out the external environment. The fence is now called a "membrane." It made possible the existence of individual living organisms. True individuals, I might add, fulfilling the criteria that professor von Weizsäcker laid out in his very broad definition of individual: "mass of matter, distinguishable from its surroundings, continuous, and of a specific form."[4] These living individuals in due time were called "cells."

Two great achievements of cells ought to be set into relief. The first, that not content with living in isolation, each one fending off as best it could the molestations of a harsh environment, they decided to found collectivities. They congregated in cooperatives, or colonies, namely the Metazoa, the first pluricellular organisms. The "primeval soup" began to look interesting: it had been augmented of croutons, as it were. Here, a division of labor was enforced that in the course of time brought forth the keen specialization of individuals: some cells were entrusted with the captation of foodstuffs, others with the digestion of the same, still others were put in charge of locomotion, communication, and so on. This led to multicellular organisms having tissues uniquely adapted for a specific function, and in due course to higher organisms with elaborate systems: muscular, digestive, circulatory, and what not. But what ought to be the chief object of reflection is the assemblage itself, the fact that an impetus to come together in mutually beneficial association should have arisen in the first place. The matter has not been pondered sufficiently.

Evolutionary history is rife with narratives of carnage, bloody struggle and rivalry. From this vantage point the world is theater of unceasing contention and merciless clash. In evolution, dog eats dog without intermittence or reprieve. "The survival of the fittest" and "the struggle for existence" are its common, widely known slogans. But when biology is re-written (for I have little doubt that biology, like every other record of human endeavor, one day will be largely rewritten), a place must be accorded to harmony and solidarity. Not all that happens is owed to ceaseless belligerence: Nature is also indebted to cooperation and peaceful agreement. Perhaps the union was of a forced kind, as with soldiers or school classmates, who come together by fate instead of choice: but for the need to survive, cells might never have developed mutual loyalty. All the same, a higher form of team-spirit emerges that lends strength to the group.

Nor does it seem to me that such words as "concord," "war," "belligerence" or "harmony" are necessarily out of place in the scientific language. Philosophy has avowed, at long last, that a so-called "objective" glance at the world is impossible. Science no longer pretends to fully impartial, perfectly indifferent or unbiased knowledge. We have learned that to us, human beings, the world is never neutral. The objects of reality we must apprehend as helpful or unhelpful, beneficial or deleterious, agreeable or repellent, pleasant or unpleasant, dangerous or reassuring. This we simply cannot avoid. Hence, an uncolored, absolutely equanimous cognition of reality, is one more ideal that we must do without. This, too, will have to be re-written one day.

The second great achievement of cells, to which we owe our very existence, was the invention of sexual reproduction. Mark its momentous, transcendent importance. Until then, cells had done well by simple fission. So well, that it could be said truthfully that the individual cell was "virtually immortal," since when threatened by senescence and death it simply split into two new beings identical to itself. Else it might be said that reproduction and death were to unicellular organisms one and the same thing (since splitting into two the parent ceases to be its former self, and therefore dies), whereas in higher animals these life-milestones are always separate.

Be that as it may, it must be owned that asexual reproduction, with its simplistic "copy and cut" program, worked excellently well. Bacteria have reproduced in this manner, with a success that needs no reemphasis. Many plants reproduce by forming offshoots that separate and grow independently. So do some multicellular animals, like *Hydra*. Flatworms pinch in the middle, then divide, and each half regenerates the missing half. Even when individuals have differentiated into male and female, sexual reproduction may be used sparingly, or not at all. Among some rotifers ("wheel animalcules") and water fleas, males are unknown: females reproduce without mating (parthenogenesis) giving rise to females only. Then, it is not as if there were no alternative ways: there is hermaphroditism, and the peculiar form of reproduction known as "gynogenesis," in which male and female exist, and the male produces sperm, but this does not unite with the female cell: it merely 'activates' the egg, prodding it, so to speak, into further development.

Nor can it be maintained that asexual reproduction is always disadvantageous in evolution. Generally speaking, the same package of genes is handed down from generation to generation; but, after, all, it is a set of genes already proven useful in bestowing hardihood to its possessors. Species of freshwater rotifers are known that have propagated by generation of females only, and done so successfully for the last forty million years. "A long time to go without sex," comments wryly a scientist alluding to this fact, while letting it be understood that the perdurability of at least some species is none the worse for the protracted deprivation.[5]

Why, then, did sexual reproduction come into being? Higher animals stick to this practice with unyielding tenacity. Bees do it, birds do it, proclaims the popular expression; and vertebrates, pontificate biologists, *all* do it. Some say Nature resorted to this as an expedient to accumulate beneficial mutations,—that is to say, genes helpful in coping with an adverse, rapidly changing environment. By blending the genomes of different individuals, the winning combination is likelier to result; and once this would spread in the population, the vitality of the race would be enhanced. Others counter that this is not so; that most mutations are bad, anyway; and that Nature's main preoccupation was to get rid of harmful mutations. During mating, the parents' genes are sorted, and some of the offspring are bound to get a whole load of bad genes; others, more fortunate, a higher share of the good. The former are unfit to survive and are eliminated; the latter go on living and propagate. "Survival of the fittest?" Some seem to think that Nature's grand design is to produce the race of the *Übermensch*. Evolutionary concepts may be clad in fascist attire without incurring blame.

I like to imagine that the invention of sexual reproduction came about as an offshoot of the ruthless cell-eats-cell culture of the pre-Cambrian geologic age. Predator cells probably ate some of the losers, and genes of the ingested inserted into the genome of the ingesting, as interiorized genes are wont to do. Merging with each other, from attempts at mutual cannibalism, became the vogue. The result was so invigorating, that the motto of the survivors soon became "Let copulation thrive," as *King Lear* would exclaim billions of years later (in act VI, vi,114).

What constrained us to be two in order to generate one? For if we consider alternative possibilities, the question could be "Why two"? Why is it that two must get together to procreate? Why not three, four or five? Think how many more interesting French novels might have been produced if our normal method of mating had required group sex! And what a boon for lawyers, psychologists, geneticists, anthropologists, and others! But most of us are inclined to believe that matters are complicated enough as they are, and do not relish greater embroilment for the sake of enhanced scholarly production. We are content to accept biology as it is, and if there is a hidden plan or an intention behind the observable phenomena, we must realize it escapes all physical means of investigation. It falls within the realm of myth and religion.

The Pythagoreans, who saw the ineffable essence of the universe reflected in mathematics and geometry, believed in a mystical basis for sexual reproduction. They saw something magic and preternatural in the triangle, hence a superior harmony in the number three. It seemed to them preordained that the participants in generation should be three: the one who generates, the one who carries the gestation, and the one who is engendered.

Count Buffon (1707-1788) in his *Histoire Naturelle*, recalls the Pythagorean belief, for which the succession of individuals in a species is but the fleeting image of the changeless, eternal harmony of the triangle, which is "universal prototype of all existence and all the generations: that is why two individuals were needed to produce a third one. That is what constitutes the essential order of father and mother, and the relationship to the son."[6] Our modern technology has transformed the Pythagorean magic triangle into various polyhedrons, less pure in design and, no doubt, less auspicious. But the corrupting of this geometry falls out of our purview at this juncture.

Functional specialization in multicellular organisms went hand in hand with change of shape. Cells in charge of conducting nervous impulses grew long, stringy extensions like

electric lines, or entangled fibers with branchings and cross-
ings, like the wires in a switchboard. Cells in charge of
absorption developed canal systems, and innumerable folds
that augmented the absorptive surface. Shape modification in
reproductive cells was spectacular. These cells are, properly
speaking, the "germs" (from Latin *germen*, seed, offshoot,
twig, and later offspring), a term inappropriately restricted in
popular usage to bacteria or to infective microorganisms.

Compared to cells in the rest of the body, the male and
female germs were modified in ways that seem aberrant,
unexampled, and almost monstrous. Their mutual disparity
reached into the grotesque. The male germ-cell was reduced
to mere vehicle for the transmission of the father's genes: its
nucleus elongated, ellipsoid, tapered at the tip, bullet-like,
prepared for advance and incursion, and loaded with DNA
that was tightly packed for ease of transport. As to its cytoplasm, it was practically eliminated, so that the male germ is
unencumbered by the numerous organelles of regular cells.
Behind the nucleus was placed a long, flexible tail, the fla-
gellum, to propel the spermatozoon (a misnomer, since it is
not an animalcule, a *zoon*, even though the tadpole appearance suggested to early microscopists an organized animal)
toward the egg-cell, the oocyte or ovocyte (also a misnomer,
since it is not a little egg). Thus provided, the male germ
could move fast, and did so tirelessly, with fluttering, waving,
spasmodic, and whip-lash motions of its tail.

As the male germ-cell is the smallest of cells in the body,
the female germ is the largest. A hundred times, and in some
species a thousand times larger than its male counterpart.
Enormous, obese, weighed down by a surfeit of reserves. For

all that the male is feverish, jittery, subsultory, and always tossing and turning, the female germ is languorous, torpid, slow-paced, held down by a massive body full of nutrients. I am reminded of a haunting, nightmarish vision of a writer influenced by the surrealist movement, the Argentinian J. Rodolfo Wilcox (1919-1978), who emigrated to Italy after a considerable body of work in Spanish, and continued a distinguished literary career in the language of his adoptive country. Wilcox describes an imaginary being, a fantastic animal that could be born only from the fertile, overflowing, and somewhat intimidating life-force that gave rise to the female germ.

The oneiric vision presents us with a gigantic beast called "Ermeta" (was Wilcox alluding to the "hermetic," inexplicable nature of the creature? He does not say). She is a kind of sow lying lazily in her lair, in a grotto that traps the humid heat of a landscape that we tend to imagine tropical. Hairy as she is, she flaunts a hairless belly furnished with two rows of symmetrically disposed nipples. Milling around these is her brood, the many little ones that push each other, climb on each other, saunter and roll around, and insist until they fall asleep, satiated, on their mother's thighs. Ermeta lies still, eyes closed, but she hardly sleeps; often, the pains appear and she goes into labor. All she does is to bring young to the world. Between parturitions she comes out of the cave and eats a little, munching in a hurry amidst the noisy, stridulous whines of her young, that push, and tussle, and tumble, and bite each other's tender tails, until their mother comes, who, with an expert push of her muzzle aligns them in strict correspondence with her teats—of which she has twenty-four.

Ermeta returns to her slumber, waiting for the pains of the next labor. How many young does she have? She does not know. She cannot count, for she has little in the way of cerebral gray matter: "just enough to bring forth a numerous family into the world, which is almost nothing," writes Wilcox.[7] But in exchange she has a splendiferous, tense, rounded belly, well adorned with a double row of dugs. An abdomen that trembles with each sigh that she exhales, and which confers on her a majestic, imposing air.

The ample, generous, overflowing constitution of the female germ-cell has important consequences for inheritance. Germ-cells, both male and female, have only half the number of chromosomes of other bodily cells (they lose the missing half by a process known as *meiosis*, or reductional division). The two parent germs fuse together at the start of sexual reproduction, and, as the respective nuclei come together, each contributes one-half of the chromosomes to the new being that is conceived, the *zygote*. The striking difference in size of the male and female germs notwithstanding, their nuclei have the same number of chromosomes (twenty-three each), and their respective contributions to the conceptus are equivalent. The fertilized egg, the zygote, therefore will have received one-half of its genes from the father, and one-half from the mother.

All these are well known facts, that even those of us who are old learned at school. What the older generation did not learn at school, because it is knowledge of more recent acquisition, is that there is a second set of genes that resides not in the nucleus, but in the cell's *mitochondria*, the cytoplasmic organelles in charge of producing most of the energy derived from the breakdown of lipids and sugars. These subcellular structures possess their own DNA, which is different from the DNA in the nucleus (for one thing, instead of the "classic" double helix disposed in long, tightly packed strands, it is arrayed in circles, like rings; moreover, the entire molecule is functional, whereas in nuclear DNA there are segments that function as genes and "silent" stretches without presently known function), and spells out the synthesis of proteins that are found nowhere but in mitochondria.

In sum, there is a second genomic system, and this unique genome is entirely of maternal origin. It matters not whether the newly generated being is male or female: its mitochondrial genome comes exclusively from the mother. In all of us it came from our mother, who received it from her mother, who in turn had it from her mother, and so on, until we reach the Mother of Us All, the "Mitochondrial Eve," a hypothetical (and controversial) female who lived in Africa over 200,000 years ago.[8]

It could not have been otherwise. The spermatozoon is reduced to a nucleus laden with DNA, and a tail to propel it forward. It could hardly be expected to contribute much cytoplasm to the conceptus, when itself carries but a thin sheath to cover its own nakedness: just enough to ensure its survival without hindering its jactitation. When it penetrates the female germ-cell it delivers as much genetic material, *i.e.*, as many genes or chromosomes, as does the female parent. The child is truly "bipartisan," it has as many reasons to think itself descended from the father, as from the mother. But the second genomic system comes from the mother, and from the mother only. These genes, as far as is known, do not contribute directly to shape the hereditary characteristics of the offspring; and are not subject to a Mendelian pattern of inheritance. The mitochondrial genes form barely 1%-2% of the total genome of an individual. But it is unavoidable to think that they must influence somehow the development of the conceptus in a very important way. What good are the best paternal genes, if they are to be immersed in a sickly cellular milieu, poisoned by sundry toxic products of a defective cytoplasm? This milieu is maternal almost in its entirety.

There is much that must yet be learned about the ways in which the maternal germ-cell contribution influences embryonic development. However, the people did not need much scientific sophistication to perceive that the role of the mother must be paramount in this regard. De Quincey, in his biographical essay on Shakespeare, voiced this popular sentiment:

> "It is certain that no great man has ever existed, but that his greatness has been rehearsed and predicted in one or the other of his parents. And it cannot be denied that in the most eminent men, where we have had the means of pursuing the investigation, the mother has more frequently been repeated and reproduced than the father. We have known cases where the mother has furnished all the intellect, and the father all the moral sensibility, upon which assumption the wonder ceases that Cicero, Lord Chesterfield, and other brilliant men, who took the utmost pains with their sons, should have failed so conspicuously; for possibly the mothers had been women of excessive and even exemplary stupidity."[9]

Thus, the billions of cells of which we are made can be assigned to one of only two kinds: a large, complex family that constitutes bodily structures in all their diversity (bone, skin, muscle, nerve, etc.), and another line of cells whose function is exclusively reproductive (sperm and ovum). The former is "somatic," since it constitutes the *soma* or body; the latter is the "germ" cell line. For a long time it was assumed that the germ produces a soma, which produces a germ, which itself produces another soma, and so on indefinitely. Not so, pronounced a German professor by the name of August Weismann (1834-1914). The germ, he said, is not formed by the soma in which it happens to be enclosed, but derives from the preceding germ.

Weismann, physician and student of zoology, loved microscopy, and would have liked to concentrate on a field requiring much peering through the microscope. A disease of the eyes toppled his youthful dreams. He still worked in a laboratory, but much of his work was strictly "armchair research." A result of his cogitations was the theory of the "continuity of *germ plasm*," which he formulated in 1883, and published shortly thereafter.[10] The germ plasm, he proposed, was the genetic material, the substance in which resided the characteristics that parents transmit to their offspring. Furthermore, he proposed that this material existed in the cell's nucleus, not in the cytoplasm, as was then believed, and was passed on intact from generation to generation. (In broad terms he was right: today the "germ plasm" would be the nuclear DNA).

In Weismann's view, very early in the formation of an embryo a class division is established: most cells will go on to form the embryo's body (somatic cells), but a few are set aside, or as it became customary to say, "segregated." The latter class of cells constitute the germ-cell line or germinal cells: to them, and to them alone, belongs the exalted mission of perpetuating the species. They are the bearers of the "germ plasm," which is carefully and exactingly handed down, like a precious heirloom, from one generation to the next. With obvious partiality for his own theory (how true it is that the creatures of the intellect may enjoy as great or greater preferment than the issue of flesh-and-blood), Weismann affirmed that the whole purpose of the life of the species is to maintain the integrity of the "germ plasm." Flaunting no little philosophical disinvolture, he postulated that our bodies are mere tools for the preservation of the "germ plasm": the somatic cells simple trustees, as it were, of the germ-cell line.

As it turned out, the theory had consequences that could be called revolutionary in its day. Mark the implications. The father, grandfather and great-grandfather were dedicated athletes and impressive muscle-men; still, the son turns out to be a weakling. This is because muscle-building, since it affects only the somatic cells, is not hereditary. To use another example: you amputate the tail of a mouse (I assume for the moment that you have the nerve for this sort of truculence. The example is canonical, and not imaginary: the described experiment was actually performed by Weismann and others), and that of its offspring. Then, you continue lopping off murine tails, litter after litter, for twenty or fifty generations of abused mice. It does not matter how far you push your obduracy and how long you perform this unfeeling experiment: the next generation of mice will be tailed. In other words, acquired features are not inheritable, since they do not involve the germ-cell line. There is no point in saying that we apply our efforts to develop skills or aptitudes (and enjoin our children and grandchildren to do the same) so that these dexterities will slowly grow to perfection in our descendants. We do not perfect the race by our own volition: it is all in the hands of the forces of evolution, which are Olympianly disdainful of our yearnings and aspirations.

Now then, we find ourselves provided with a rich array of somatic cells, and a highly *sui generis* strain of cells, the germinal cells. We are ready to reproduce. What next? We come up against the striking realization that, under normal conditions of biology, each one of us has only one-half of the reproductive apparatus. Procreation imposes the inescapable necessity of finding the missing half. This biologic reality lends an undying charm to the well known Greek myth, expounded by Aristophanes in Plato's *Symposium* or *Banquet* (189c-193a).

Mankind, the myth says, was originally very different from what it now is. For one thing, the shape of the human body was spheroidal, but people could run at great speed, rolling about like tumble weeds. Each person had one head with two faces looking in opposite directions, four hands, four arms and four legs, of marvelous assistance in their displacements. Their genitals were also double, and of three possible kinds: male, female, and a combination of the two. Again the magic triangle! Why three? Aristophanes gives us a reason as good as any: "because the sun, the earth and the moon are three," and men were descended from the sun, women came from the earth, and the bisexual race, or Androgynous race, from the moon.

The original mankind wished to imitate the gods, of

whom they thought themselves worthy rivals. Their imperti-
nence irritated Zeus, who in punishment decided to cut them
in two, "like a sorb-apple which is halved for pickling," so as
to reduce their strength, and increase their numbers in servitude. Zeus wished not to annihilate them, but to weaken
them. The plane of section was quickly repaired. Apollo did
a nice job of reconstruction, smoothed out the folds, and
drew in the skin like a purse-string at the region now corresponding to the belly, ending the closure with a tight knot in
what is now the navel.

Since then, each half goes through life desperately seeking
its complementary half. The sons of the original men look for
fulfillment with another man (I gather in ancient Greece this
lineage must have been no small segment of the population),
for only the homosexual union restitutes the original complete man in all his virility. The female descendants of primeval
woman are the lesbians, who strive to find the right woman;
and the posterity of the Androgynous searches for a complement in a person of the opposite sex. Thus, the yearning that
lovers experience for each other relates to this, that both wish
to come together in a reconstruction of the ancestral type;
and the tight embraces in which they hold one another
express the undying impetus that propels them to reconstruct
the original Unity.

Is this really the message that Plato left us on the nature
of the erotic? Not at all. In the *Banquet*, Aristophanes develops with gusto this idea, that love is a nostalgia for the lost
unity; that we go through life looking for our lost half, this
"double" of ourselves, to which we yearn to adhere every bit
of our persons—as if we were forcefully sticking our bodies

against our own specular image, in a desperate attempt at completing the totality that we once were. Love, in this view, is at bottom defect, lack, incompleteness. But, contrary to this arresting myth, the true nature of love is explicated by Diotima, after warning her hearers that they may not be prepared to understand it (*Banquet* 210a). Love, they are told, is a divine revelation, a state of possession by supernatural forces, during which the deity is revealed to the lovers, enabling them to "engender in beauty."

Therefore love implies procreation or engendering: it is not incompleteness, but surfeit. At the physical level, this means the generation of offspring; on a spiritual plane, the production of art, beauty, or works of the intellect. Jean-Pierre Vernant[11] put it marvelously in stating that the Aristophanic formula of the erotic was $1/2 + 1/2 = 1$, whereas the Platonic one said $1 + 1 = 3$. Two lovers, two separate individualities come together to create a third one. Unconventional arithmetic realized by the epiphany of a divinity for which love was not a lack, but an abundance of realizable potential.

Believe only the Delivery

RABELAIS DERIDED THE MALE'S HESITATION TO SETTLE down. In the Third Book of *Pantagruel,* which Anatole France believed to be the most beautiful and most replete with delightful comicity of the *Pantagruel* books,[1] the "wise buffoon" represented his personage, Panurge, worried from seeing his youth slip away, and thinking of marriage. Should he marry? Should he not? He consults his teacher, Pantagruel, and an amusing consultation follows.

"It is generally advantageous to marry," says the pupil. The mentor agrees, and advises him to do it.

"But assuming it were disadvantageous," rejoins the student, "it were better not to do it." The master agrees again: "In that case don't do it."

"Then, of course," adds Panurge, "life must be faced without a companion, which is a harsh thing to do." To which Pantagruel replies: "Then marry, in the name of God!"

Upon which, Panurge counter-argues: "But if my wife made me a cuckold, a living species that, as is well known to

you, has of late proliferated abundantly in this country . . ."
And Pantagruel: "Then do not marry, if you are afraid to
receive retribution for your past deeds."

And Panurge: "Right. But if I were to be united to an
honest, lovely and virtuous woman . . . ? And Pantagruel:
"Marry then!"

The consultation prolongs itself in this pendular fashion,
exploited by comedy writers in the Middle Ages, and later
imitated by Molière. There are reasons to marry, and there
are reasons not to marry.

Panurge and Pantagruel decide to consult the forces of
the occult for an answer. They resort first to divinatory arts:
stick a pin three times in a volume of Virgil or Homer, and see
the words on which the pin was stuck. Unfortunately, the
words thus chosen form pure gibberish: nothing can be concluded. Next, they place their trust in the interpretation of
dreams, but this expedient is equally ineffective. One of the
dreams, however, is quite suggestive: Panurge dreams that he
is married, and his wife caresses him in many ways, after
which she hangs on his head a pair of horns. Having decided
that all these signs are inconclusive (a recalcitrant optimist!),
the next step is to consult a Sibyl, then another seer, then a
philosopher, and still other possible sources of good counsel.
In the end, tired, seeing that there is no firm, reasoned answer,
Panurge impatiently decides for marriage on a sudden
impulse.

This is the way things go, and although the times have
changed, the male's motivations have remained surprisingly
unchanged in many societies. Many are afraid that, in the
event their wives are disloyal, their posterity will not be truly

theirs. Wrote Francisco de Quevedo, the incomparable master satirist of Spain's Golden Century:

> "If paternity were to be investigated there would be a confusion of 'here hand-me-my-firstborn-rights, and there take-your-inheritance.' In the matter of bellies there is a lot to be said, and since babies are made in the dark, with no light, no one can tell who was conceived by full individual quota, or who by partial fee [as in purchases by many payors], and it is best to believe the delivery, for thus all of us are heirs, without dispute [. . .] How many think you on Judgement Day shall recognize their father in their page, their squire, their slave and their neighbor, and how many fathers shall find themselves childless? There you shall see that!"[2]

What is a woman to do, in the face of this male preoccupation with the exclusivity of sex and generation? For one thing, men make it difficult for womankind: they do everything in their power to make women surrender, and then become incensed because they obtained a surrender. A more childish, irrational and contradictory attitude would be hard to find. Sor Juana Inés de la Cruz (1651-1695), the celebrated nun and eximious Mexican poet, pointed out the absurdity of those "Foolish Men Who Accuse [women]" (the title of her best known poem), and who resemble *Al niño que pone el coco / Y luego le tiene miedo* ('The child who invents a bugbear / And then grows afraid of it").

The puerility of the situation would be simply laughable, if it did not sometimes cloak itself with the bloody mantle of tragedy. The obsession with Woman's innocence strains credibility. In the past in many societies, and today in some, "purity," in the sense of complete absence of premarital experience with sexual relations, is expected of her. Not only expected, but demanded with fierce, uncompromising obstinacy.

The problem of how to detect an infringement of the rules was pondered by men with patience and meticulousness worthy of loftier goals. Would the loss of purity be manifest in her carriage, her gestures or her demeanor? No, since she is an expert at dissembling. It is not in vain that her name is Eve, and according to a medieval tradition, *Eva* , her Latin appelation, is an ellipsis of *Extra* *vada*, "go out," reflecting the divine repudiation that she suffered when expelled from Paradise on account of her misconduct. (A second version is equally unflattering: *Eva* is an inversion of *Ave*, the Latin "Hail"; and just as the latter was used to wish health and salvation on those greeted, the former, being inverted, indicates that women are the cause of ills and perdition for men).[3] But if she is too smart to be detected by attention to evanescent or impermanent details, men's obsession found a better mark, a piece of evidence that they were willing to trust: the hymen.

Curious to remark, the very existence of the hymeneal membrane, on whose account so much sound and fury have been spent, was for centuries a matter of debate. There is an illustrious tradition of learned men, from ancient Greek philosophers to French *encyclopédistes* of the Enlightenment, who affirmed that the hymen was a figment of the imagination. Not ignorant men, but famous physicians and anatomists, men who practiced dissections, were disbelievers. Ambroise Paré was of the opinion that the diagnosis of vir-

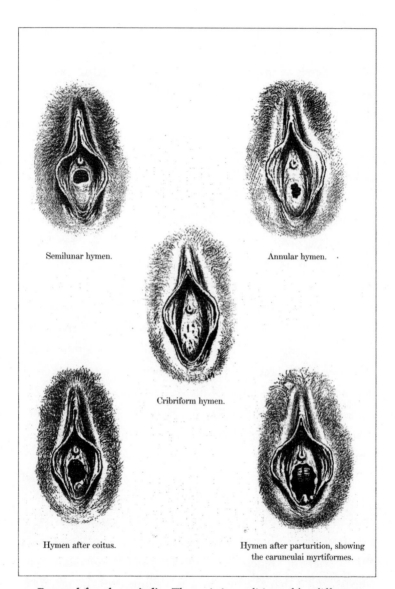

Semilunar hymen.

Annular hymen.

Cribriform hymen.

Hymen after coitus.

Hymen after parturition, showing the carunculai myrtiformes.

External female genitalia. The artist's rendition of he different types of hymen reflects in its detailed meticulousness the male preoccupation with the anatomical mark of virginity.

(*From Blair Bell, 1919*)

ginity, or of the loss of the same, was impossible to establish by examination of the genital region. As to the hymen, it simply did not exist:

> "To determine whether or not a girl is a maiden is quite difficult; nevertheless, the matrons give it for certain that they can know this, for they say they find a rupture in a membrane that tears on the first sexual encounter [*une taie qui se rompt au premier combat vénérique*]. But I have formerly shown in my book *On Generation*, chapter 50, that in twenty thousand women one finds not one such membrane."[4]

In the seventeenth century, a French physician, Nicolas Venette (1633-1698), believed that the hymen was a postmortem formation. He wrote: ". . . after death it sometimes happens that Nature being willing to preserve the womb of some tender woman, produces a membrane below the urinary passage that air or other exterior matters may not disorder the interior parts; and this membrane is properly called hymen, or the true maidenhead."[5] Why would Nature wish to preserve the "interior parts" of a dead person, Venette did not explain.

Debate as to the existence of the hymen continued up to the beginning of the present century. Auguste Debay, prolific, highly popular author (now mostly unread) and sexologist *avant la lettre* at the close of the nineteenth century, denied, like Paré, the normal presence of a hymen or of visible marks of defloration. His denial was emphatic, albeit clothed in the affectedly cavalier tone of a Parisian fashionable of *la belle époque*:

"Anatomists who admit [the existence of] the hymen say that its tear produces, after cicatrization, little buds to which they gave the coquettish name of '*myrtiform caruncles*.' The truth is that physicians [. . .] have only rarely perceived such a membrane. In contrast, they have seen wrinkles, rugosities, eminences, furrows, folds of the vaginal membrane, more or less effaced depending on the woman's legal status, that is, whether maiden or married; but they saw nothing that might resemble myrtles."[6]

Contemporary medicine reaffirms the existence of the hymen. It is a fold of the vaginal mucosa situated at the entrance of the vaginal orifice, says *Gray's Anatomy*, the inner edges of which are normally in contact with each other, so that the orifice appears as a cleft between them. And various texts still repeat, although rather sparingly, the lore dear to anatomists of the past: that it may look like a half-moon; or a ring broadest posteriorly; or a middle membranous strip flanked by spaces on each side; or a sieve, ("cribriform") pierced by numerous little holes; or a complete occluding septum that must be incised to secure the egress of menses; or the swinging panels of an old-fashioned saloon door; and so on. *Gray's Anatomy* admonishes: "It may persist after copulation, so that its presence cannot be considered a sign of virginity."[7]

Thus, it is no longer "the seal of purity," a function that its ancient Latin name, *signaculum*, seal, used to denote. Nor has this impeded the appearance of articles in the medical literature, purporting to illustrate the effects of defloration; for physicians who may be called upon as expert witnesses in

forensic proceedings dealing with such crimes as rape or sexual abuse of minors, ought to be cognizant of the anatomic
injuries sustained by the victims.

In some human societies, the blood-stained bed sheets are
publicly displayed after the wedding night, as a proclamation
that the bride reached the nuptial bed in the state of immac-
ulateness demanded by local tradition. I was a pubescent boy
when I first heard of this barbaric ritual, whose description I
found quite mortifying. The gentleness and poetry of first
love seemed rudely supplanted by images of bloody violence.
That the sweet beloved should be seen in the guise of a
besieged fortress to be taken by assault, was bad enough. But
that a most intimate act should be denigrated by violence,
and its marks then put up for all to see, was adding shame to
injury.

Yet, ours is a violent world: behind a thin veneer of civi-
lization, the raw impulses and barbaric tendencies survive
intact. Admixed with the noblest inflowings of the spirit of
men's love, is the atavic impetus of rape: the stone-age drive
to possess a woman by force. According to Giulia Sisa, the
ancient Greek poetry of *epithalamium* style, designed to be
sung by a chorus at weddings in honor of the newlyweds, was
actually intended to be sung while the newly married couple
were in their bedroom, in order to disguise the cries of pain
of the bride.[8]

Consider, then, the predicament of a young woman
caught in the chaos of the world. She comes from an exces-
sively conservative social milieu, say rural and backward, and
must contemplate the time when proof will be demanded of
her: a proof which she has reason to think she cannot furnish.

Hers is indeed a harrowing plight. Traditionally, she would seek advice from an old woman, wise in the absurd and twisted ways of men's folly. There has always been a sisterhood of old crones, who are sympathetic to young girls in trouble, provided they are of the paying kind. This ancient sorority is composed of females who are a little of everything: healers, go-betweens, and seers or witches. Dante called them, I think without good reason, "sad women," and assigned them, with his usual topographic specificity, to the fourth pit of the eighth circle of hell, for having ". . . cast the needle, the shuttle and the spindle, and made themselves devineresses; then wrought witchcraft with herbs and images." (*Vedi le triste che lasciaron l'ago la spola e il fuso, e fecersi indovine; fecer malie con erbe e con imago.* Canto XX, 121-123).

In their infernal abode these "sad" women are strangely conformed: their heads are reversed, the face turned to the back, which forces them always to walk backwards, in punishment, Dante tells us, of their impudent pretension to guess the future, and thus to "see" forward in time. These reverse-headed women constantly weep; and, as the poet tells us in a deliberately coarse, yet striking image, their tears bathe their buttocks, rolling down along the sides of the intergluteal fissure.

In the Spanish-speaking world, such an old woman is a *celestina*. The name comes from a novel, a classic work in Spanish letters that first appeared in the Castilian city of Burgos in 1499, entitled *The Comedy of Calisto and Melibea,* written by Fernando de Rojas (1465-1541). Despite the title, it is not a comedy, but a tragedy of ill-starred lovers, whose passion brings them, and their associates, to a violent end. Although one may have expected two young lovers, the chief protagonists in a classic novel, to be enshrined in the popular imagination, the truth is that they quickly slinked into oblivion. In contrast, a secondary personage, Celestina, became immortal thanks to the lively, masterful character depiction by the novelist.

She received the extraordinary homage that is to pass into the language as a common word. In effect, a *celestina* came to mean a match-maker, a go-between, an *alcahueta*. The latter term connotes rather a procurer. Not in the pristine sense of this word, meaning an attorney who intercedes in our favor and transacts our businesses, (a meaning retained in the Spanish *procurador*; fr. Latin *procurare*: *pro*: for, on behalf of, and *curare*, to take care), but in today's most common acceptation of the term: "one who makes it a trade to obtain women for the satisfaction of lust." This is what she is, and she might have been something worse before, since a preacher of centuries past sonorously declaimed that "Strumpets in their Youth turn Procurers in their Age." Be that as it may, Celestina was elevated to the category of a Spanish archetype, in the company of icons of worldwide renown: *Don Quijote* the idealist, impractical dreamer, *Don Juan* the philanderer and irredeemable sinner, and *Celestina* the bawd, a female procurer or procuress.

She is much more than that, however. Which is why our disconsolate girl seeks her advice. We can picture the unfortunate young lady entering timidly into Celestina's dark shop, at night, to be sure that no one sees her. She looks around her timorously, and discovers all sorts of objects on the shelves. There are unguents, and essences for the bath; hair dyes that the old woman makes from vine shoots, oak leaves, alum, saltpeter and other ingredients; and powders for the face, composed with senna pods, tarragon, and what not. There are nostrums and medicines for the ills peculiar to women. There are preparations allegedly helpful to reinvigorate a flagging virility, and others—much less frequently pressed into service—which, it is rumored, can punish by foisting a droopy flaccidity upon a virility grown too arrogant and overbearing. For, let's face it. Celestina has more than a little of the witch in her. Therefore it is not surprising to find flasks containing parts of the body of birds that are easily ensnared. The theory, dear to magicians of all times, is that a part of an object preserves and communicates the virtues and faults of the whole. And since a bird that does not escape the traps of the hunter is by nature stupid, slow or confused, its parts should be especially fit to enter into the composition of love potions, for the lovesick are, by definition, stupefied, crazed, and reduced to imbecility.

In the back of the shop, on a dark cupboard, the young lady will spot some of Celestina's most carefully guarded possessions. At first sight, they seem to be trivial objects: a packet of very thin furriers' needles wrapped in delicate paper; some lengths of very fine, waxed silken thread; and some medicinal plants. Nothing especially exotic or unusual. But with these simple tools, Celestina worked miracles: she restored the lost virginity to those women who requested it. Her biographer, Fernando de Rojas, tells us that thanks to this admirable dexterity she sold to the French ambassador— whose attentiveness seems to have lagged behind his sexual appetite—three times the same girl for a virgin!

The restitution of the lost maidenhead was no less than a miracle. Medieval theologians quoted Saint Jerome as saying: "I shall speak boldly: although God can do anything, He cannot make a virgin of a girl who no longer is one. He certainly has the power to free her from her distress, but not to restore the crown of her lost virginity to her."[9] Jerome avoided blasphemy by adding that if God cannot accomplish a particular act, it is only because He does not wish to do so. And He does not wish to reconstitute a vanished virginity, because, in His supreme wisdom, He has decided to impress upon the mind of the deflowered woman that what she lost as a thing of little value, she is never going to recover, try as she might with bitterest remorse and penitence. The fallen woman shall then be forced to keep ever present in her mind the marks of her error, with the ensuing contrition and pangs of conscience being most salutary for her soul.

What divine Providence could not, or would not accomplish, Celestina did, if the price was right. But what if a modern physician, at the dawn of the twenty-first century, should be requested to perform this service? This situation is not rare.

In the large cities of the industrialized world live many immigrants that bring with them unyielding ancestral customs. They also harbor such irrational attitudes as the deeply felt conviction that a woman may be put to death if she is believed to be promiscuous. In the least enlightened parts of the Islamic world, but not only there, this horrible deed has been known to be carried out by the brothers, uncles, or even the father of the allegedly guilty woman. Where tribal customs are deeply rooted in society, the murderers may escape prosecution, even if the law decrees their act punishable. In the industrialized West, murder under these circumstances is not likely to pass unpunished. But if not murder, then shame, rancor, financial loss, a broken engagement, and ill will between families, will inevitably occur. Imagine yourself being a physician who is consulted by a teary-eyed damsel in distress. Will you not, as physician, repair a torn hymen and avoid so much woe?

The operation itself is no surgical prowess. It is quite simple, which is why Celestina could do it well, much to the benefit of her local fame. Technically, it is called "hymenorrhaphy," and consists of shaving off the surface epithelium that has grown over the edges of the tear, then approximating the remnants of the hymen, and suturing them together. The procedure is performed under local anesthesia, and, if properly performed, is quite safe. In the Arab world, Egypt was recently said to have become the center for hymernorrhaphies, where women in need of this operation flock from all the Arab countries, far and near, and pay between one hundred and six hundred U.S. dollars to have it performed.[10] Like other illegal operations, hymenorrhaphies are performed in a variety of circumstances, safe and unsafe, in clinics or in private houses.

A refinement that recalls the cleverness of Celestina and the ribald stories of Brantôme, consists in suturing to the repaired tissue a capsule containing a blood-like fluid: on the wedding night the capsule will burst, the fluid will ooze, and the bridegroom will be utterly persuaded that his bride was a virgin. Which is proof that there is nothing new under the sun, and that the boundless stupidity of men can be counted on, who are prompt to overvalue what they do not know, what matters not, and what they can never corroborate, anyway.

The Egyptian Medical Association declared itself against this operation. Al Azhar, Egypt's highest religious body, also condemns the operation, branding it contrary to the laws of the Koran, which lay it down that the bride must be a virgin. But the Egyptian police force is not so sweepingly condemnatory: policemen suspect that the operation has reduced the rate of murders inspired by a perceived sullying of men's honor. "There is no ill that does not come for some good," says an old Spanish proverb.

In Holland, it has been legal for the patient to remove and destroy all the notes in the medical record. Thus, after the operation no inculpatory material evidence remains. Reportedly, the women who benefit from these practices have no regrets.[11] Some physicians have argued that it is unethical for a professional to perform a surgical operation on social grounds alone, without true medical indication; that by doing this the physician is guilty of collusion and deceit; and that a medical doctor also has responsibilities toward the bridegroom, or the families involved. Others counter that the question of deceit does not pose itself; that the operation is intended for the benefit of the woman only; and that the procedure ought to be accorded the confidentiality due to a patient-doctor relationship, in keeping with an ancient and noble tradition of medical practice. Above all, it would be rash to disregard the fact that the patient is at risk of violent reprisal, and that the operation greatly reduces the odds of this taking place.

One might have thought that this kind of ethical dilemma would no longer pose itself in a world preoccupied by momentous biomedical quandaries, such as cloning, the definition of life, and the nature of personal identity. But in the realm of human affairs we can expect anything, save pre-dictability and consistency.

The male obsession with the "purity" of his wife and the legitimacy of his heirs has very deep roots in history and psy-chology. It is especially intriguing that this obsession has been as vehement and enduring as it is illogical and absonant to nature. These are also the qualities that make it an easy tar-get for satire. Quevedo felt that in Judgement Day many will realize that their ancestry, or their offspring, is not exactly what they thought it was. We may not have to wait that long. He could not have known that the powerful tools of molecu-lar biology today can exclude or confirm alleged paternity with astounding accuracy. DNA analysis is used with increas-ing frequency in forensic disputes over paternity. This technol-ogy has been able to verify what popular lore long suspected, that even one of twins may be suspect. In other words, each member of a pair of twins may have a different father,[12] thus giving credence to Quevedo's assertion that "some are con-ceived '*a escote*'" (an archaic Castilian expression meaning payment of one's individual portion in a collective purchase).

Quevedo was also right in predicting that some will dis-cover their father in their slave. He could have added the cor-relative proposition: slaves may trace their genealogy to the master. Molecular genetic analysis revealed the disturbing likelihood that Thomas Jefferson fathered a son with his black slave, Sally Hemings.[13] Alas, the scientific communica-tion on Jefferson's putative offspring left little room for doubt: the technology of DNA analysis is extraordinarily accurate and sensitive. Still, the report was followed by a brisk correspondence from readers despairing to see that the great man was less than the paradigm of perfection and probity that they had imagined.

An investigation carried out in Iceland promises to be especially interesting in this regard. The Althinghi, Iceland's Parliament, recently passed a bill granting a large biotechnology company exclusive rights to build a genetic database of the entire Icelandic population. Icelanders constitute a very homogeneous group: they descend from a relatively small number of original Norse settlers, and have lived for centuries with almost no admixture, since immigration into this country has been negligible. Successive epidemics, and later the eruption of the Hekla volcano in the late 1770s, further reduced the population, and hence the genetic pool. In this genetically homogeneous human society, mutations are easy to trace. Iceland is, therefore, an excellent place to study various aspects, normal and pathologic, of human genetics. Moreover, the family histories of most individuals of this population have been computerized, for the study of genealogy has been said to be a "national obsession" here.

In this highly regimented, meticulously studied and genetically homogeneous population, the estimate has been, according to studies based on DNA analysis, that ten percent of Icelanders have a different biologic father than they thought.[14]

Of the wrath and confusion of the deceived father who dicovers the deceit, much has been said. The bewilderment of the progeny elicits relatively less commentary. But the effects of finding out that one's father is not "the same one," *i.e.*, the man one took to be one's progenitor, cannot be negligible.

In a society thoroughly suffused by the idea of a deep chasm and a moral opposition between legitimacy and illegitimacy, the bastard child is bound to suffer; little does it matter that it did nothing reprehensible: its fault is to exist. Yet, the shock of the realization is differently borne according to a number of circumstances. I am acquainted with a man whom I consider lucky for having learned of his "spurious" origin late in life. His personality was already formed: he had no problem constructing his personal identity; there was no foundational crack in his self-esteem. He knew no tortured, anxious search for a father during his most vulnerable years; no growing up with the consciousness of being somehow excluded, if not outrightly branded "a bastard," as still happens in some human groups. His mother probably did the right thing in keeping the secret as zealously as she did.

This theme is worthy of the greatest novelists. The relentless growth of doubt, the incidents that amplify it, the desperate search for evidence that confirms or denies: these are elements of a torturing passion that may, on occasion, rise to the same pitch of exasperation and despair as jealousy, hatred, envy, or any of the dismal, dark animic states that are the eternal stuff of high tragedy and drama.

Guy de Maupassant (1850-1893) has been the writer most preoccupied with the theme of illegitimate birth. His short stories or novellas have approached it from every conceivable point of view (a fact that made critics wonder whether the writer himself was troubled by doubts over the legitimacy of his own birth). Thus, in *Le Testament*, he adopts the perspective of the illegitimate child; in a later work, *L'Abandonné*, he takes the viewpoint of the child and his mother; then, in *Le Petit* and *Monsieur Parent*, that of the hoodwinked father, *i.e.*, the wrongly alleged parent; and in the gripping narrative of *Un Parricide*, the child, his parents, and society at large, all have a voice. But this writer, who is generally recognized as a superb short story teller, was going to astound his contemporaries by fashioning a classic, immortal novel, *Pierre et Jean,* centered upon an illegitimate birth.

Pierre Roland is the chief protagonist of the novel. He is the elder of two brothers in a bourgeois family. He is nervous, tenacious, intense, quite intelligent and rather moody. His brother Jean is easy going, as blond as his brother is dark, as calm as the other is excitable. Their mother, now middle aged, still keeps the traces of what used to be great physical beauty, joined to an air of distinction. The father, Mr. Roland senior, is a retired jeweler, who moves with his family from Paris to Rouen, where he can indulge to his heart's content in his favorite pastimes, boating and fishing. Nothing else interests him, and nothing troubles him. He is a man who, said Anatole France in a commentary of the novel, "attained, on first try, and quite effortlessly, the supreme wisdom."[15]

The four of them live in perfect tranquillity amidst the materialistic concerns of the bourgeoisie—which, in nineteenth century provincial France, yielded in nothing to present day's consumerism and self-centeredness—when, unexpectedly, Jean is notified that he had been named sole beneficiary in the last will of an old friend of the family, a Mr. Maréchal. This man, an old bachelor whom they used to frequent when they lived in Paris, has just died childless, leaving a large fortune in the name of Jean.

Pierre experiences some jealousy toward his fortunate brother. Nothing, however, that could not be put down to normal sibling's rivalry. Then, one evening, in the most casual way, the searing flame of his pathos is kindled. An apparently insignificant occurrence, as is not unusual, triggers the conflagration. A bar girl makes a salacious remark, to the effect that Pierre and Jean, after all, may not have the same entitlement to the inheritance. For anyone who hears the news of the bequeathal must wonder why it stipulated all for one and nothing for the other. There could be a reason for naming only one of them as legatee . . .

Pierre is incensed. The insinuation is insulting. But the barb has sunk in, and its tip is poisoned. It will not take long for the wound to fester. In effect, Jean is, unbeknownst to everyone but his mother, an adulterine bastard child.

From then on, Pierre knows no rest. He compulsively collects reasons to increase his suspicion, even while he desperately yearns not to doubt any longer. He accumulates inculpatory evidence against his mother, whom he cannot help loving dearly. He uses the cruelest subterfuges to frighten her, to punish her, to overwhelm her with the remorseful memory of her past fault. Slowly he plunges, deeper and deeper, into a hell of envy, jealousy, distrust, and alienation. In a dramatic passage that is perhaps the emotional climax of the novel, he reveals to Jean the whole truth about his origin.

Pierre's alienation could not be more thorough: from his father, who knows nothing and cares to understand nothing; from his brother, since he is the son of another man, and thus to some extent a stranger; and from his mother, because she appeared to him as deceitful. Maupassant writes:

"Yes, she had betrayed him in his tenderness, deceived him in his pious respect. She owed herself to him irreproachable, as all mothers owe themselves to their children. If the furor which possessed him reached almost to the point of hatred, it was because he sensed her more criminal toward him than toward his father.

> "The love between a man and a woman is a voluntary pact, in which the one who defaults is only guilty of perfidy; but once the woman has become a mother, her duty has increased, since Nature has entrusted her with a race. If she succumbs then, she is cowardly, unworthy, and infamous."

The reader witnesses the progressive dissolution of the ties that held together that bourgeois family, with a sense of powerlessness. For Pierre, like the other members of his family, must irrevocably precipitate toward his doom, leaving the reader with the sensation that, as with the personages of Greek tragedy, there is absolutely nothing that anyone could do to alter the inexorable accomplishment of their appointed fates.

I re-read the pages of *Pierre et Jean*, and again I must conclude that my acquaintance was lucky to have been spared the tumultuous emotions that often grip the young who discover their own bastardy. But the older man who learns that he was engendered in clandestinity or under the sign of deceit, does not fall prey to these tempestuous emotions. He knows, for one thing, that extreme reactions are almost never justified. He knows, likewise, that nothing is final or absolute; that purity itself is a relative term; that no one can claim an "innocent" birth; and that those who pretend otherwise are deceived by their own metaphors.

I am sure the biologically-minded can come up with ponderous explanations of why men insist so adamantly in making sure that their children are truly theirs. They will educe for us, most likely, some argument clothed in the raiment of evolutionary theory, about the necessity for man to spread his genes in a vertical direction, down the tree of genealogy; and timely comparisons to the behavior of males of this and that species will lend further credibility to the exposition. But apart from instinctual drives to achieve "reproductive success" (for this is the terminology in vogue), in the form of perpetuation of an individual's unique genomic constitution, I feel that men are also actuated by nostalgia. I mean a wistful desire for relations that are uncomplicated, simple, and pure. For purity or innocence is an ideal, a type of perfection that we are condemned never to reach. And how frustrating this incapacity! We were innocent one day, as children —without knowing it, of course—and cease to be so the very instant when we first become conscious of innocence. There never was a sadder fate: to have a precious thing without realizing it, and to lose it because becoming aware of its possession.

What, if not a perfervid yearning for a higher and unattainable ideal could have inspired this multisecular obsession with female virginity? But perfect purity is not within human reach. It is an ideal, that is to say an insubstantial entity, a spiritual value. Human nature is essentially alien to purity. For in us virtues must exist shaded by vices, qualities marred by defects, and uplifting impulses always alloyed with debasing inclinations.

Mark, then, the solution devised by the craftiness of men. If an ideal is unattainable, we can transform it into a thing. We can reify innocence. And just as the soul, which somehow resides in the body, was assigned by Descartes a domicile in the pineal gland, so the purity of Woman was said by men *to be* her inviolate body. Not only to coexist with her body, but to coincide with it, and more specifically with a part of her genital anatomy: the hymen. Was this not a clever solution? Once we know there is a "seal of purity," we know what to defend.

The evil of the world breeds confusion; the attacks of ill will are multi-pronged; malevolence comes at us from all sides. The saints enjoined us to cultivate the "virginity of the heart," by which they meant renunciation, self-abnegation and detachment from worldly concerns. But who can do that? If we know where to concentrate our defense, we have less to worry about. Let the enemy close in on us. We are content knowing that there is one specific object that must be defended at all costs. One only, to be preserved with all our might: the virginity of women, our Holy Grail. And then we can forget all that nonsense about the "maidenhead of the heart."

Saga of the Womb, or the
Perils of the Mother

A Many-Faced Organ

ATHENA WAS BORN FROM THE HEAD OF ZEUS; BACCHUS, from Jupiter's side (or his thigh, if you will); Buddha, from his mother's armpit, or her hip, after she was visited by a six-tusked elephant; the Yakut shamans of Siberia, from a giant fir tree that grows human embryos[1]; and a personage of an Eskimo legend, from the abdominal wall of the father, who had become pregnant by eating the mystic herring roe. All of which is well and good. But as for us, common mortals, we were born from our mother's womb. It is thus natural that we ask what sort of place might *that* be; and the answer is that, like all things in this world, it depends on the way you look at it.

To heed the usual descriptions of anatomists, our first housing is rather drab and undistinguished. It is a hollow, thick-walled muscular viscus situated in the female pelvis between the urinary bladder and the rectum: not exactly what a real estate agent would call "an exclusive neighborhood." Fully developed, but still virginal, it measures about 7.5 centimeters (about three inches) from top to bottom, some 5 centimeters in width, and 2 .5 centimeters in thickness; and it weighs between 30 and 40 grams.

An old tradition in anatomy has been to see things analogically, that is to say, to compare the mysterious organs with objects of common experience, as if the enigma could lessen in the comparison. Thus, it is common to say that the uterus is pear-shaped. But, as soon as one allows this sort of comparisons, imagination and personal idiosyncrasy begin to take over. Some will say that it looks like a gourd; others, like an inverted bottle, the narrow neck pointing downward, the widened portion above. Some anatomists compared it to an hourglass, because there is a narrow segment (isthmus) that joins its upper part, or body, and its lower portion, or neck (cervix). Hippocrates referred to it as a "vessel" or a jug (*Epidemics*, II, 6, 5).

Most often, however, the ancient Greeks saw the womb in the guise of a wineskin, and remarked with admirable acumen on the functional implications of its shape: as we purse our lips and project them forward when we suck on a straw, so does the narrow neck of the womb juts down (more avidly when stimulated by sexual desire) to draw in the male semen during coition. For when the uterus has been purgated of its monthly discharge, consequently being a bit too hot and dry, and provided it is in its normal location (for, remember, it can move!), then it will be found to be uniquely fit for drawing in the male seed. Proof, wrote Aristotle in his *Generation of Animals* (II, 4, 739b), is that pessaries, though inserted wet, are removed dry. And a modern commentator subjoins: if a bottle is heated and its neck thrust into water, as the air inside the bottle is cooled a vacuum is created, and some water will be drawn up into the neck.[2]

Pear, gourd, bottle, wineskin, jug, jar, vase, hourglass: a long list could be compiled. To one of our own contemporaries, doctor Sherwin Nuland, the image is avian.[3] For, he writes, if one can visualize the body of a bird as roughly pear-shaped (which one did he have in mind? I think of the dove of the Holy Spirit), then the extended wings are simulated by the Fallopian tubes that arise from the upper part of the body of the uterus and course outward, each accompanied by a large, broad, flattened sheet of tissue that serves to anchor the womb to the pelvic wall ("broad ligaments").

The rich unconscious symbolism of this bird-like shape or "ornithomorphism" is evident: a bird flies freely across space, and, in the elementary imagination, across time as well. So it is that magicians and shamans in primitive religions adopt a bird costume—the most favored one is the eagle—for the performance of those incantations and rituals that require them to go to "the other world."[4] A man who must transport himself to the beyond is wise to travel light. To this end, the feathered costume of a bird seems particularly well adapted. Thus, the bird-womb is unexcelled as the means of transportation that trundles newborns between the other world, that "beyond" to which we must all one day return, and our sublunary vale of tears.

The interior cavity of the womb partakes of the enigma. Its lining is a soft, velvety, pink membrane, the endometrium. Its cells enlarge greatly during pregnancy, when the entire lining membrane, now called decidua, appears swollen. Authoritative medical opinion throughout classical antiquity

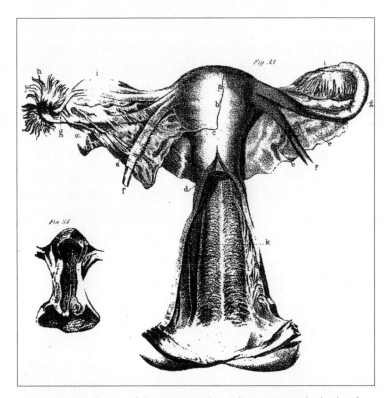

Artist's rendering of the uterus and its adnexa. From the body of the uterus emerge on each side the fallopian tubes and the structures known as broad ligaments, a conformation that has suggested the imaginative comparison with a bird and its wings. The lower part of the uterus is continuous with the vagina, whose roof has been opened to expose a ridged surface with a central white line. The inset at left shows the cavity of the uterus after removal of its anterior wall.

(Siebold, 1829)

affirmed that the uterine cavity was divided into two compartments, right and left. This idea may have originated in analogy to the testicles of the male. Or perhaps early observers, having seen the fallopian tubes emerging on each side of the uterus, imagined the latter's interior to be duplex. This misconception of the ancients is well known: embryos developing in the right-sided compartment would be male; those gestated in the left-sided chamber turned into females. Preposterous as it might seem, this fallacy was less vaulting than the medieval belief that the uterus was subdivided into seven cells: three on the right for the males, three on the left for females, and one in the center for hermaphrodites.[5]

The doctrine of seven cells in the uterine cavity may have been derived from an ancient belief according to which the number of compartments in the womb corresponded to the maximum number of embryos that could be borne at one time. Alternatively, it could have arisen by analogy to the number of mamillae in certain animals (like the sow, which has seven on each side), since it was common at the time to transpose anatomical and physiological concepts derived from observations in animals, directly to humans. Scholars believe that esoteric ideas from the Neo-Pythagorean, Neo-Platonic, and Hermetic literature, by imparting a mystical aura to the number seven, may have contributed to strengthen belief in seven uterine chambers. There was no dearth of this esoterica adverting to the somatic sphere: it takes seven days for the semen to turn to flesh; the menstrual flow normally lasts seven days; the age of man is seven decades; seven-month fetuses are viable (whereas those of eight months, it was held, were not); there are seven orifices in the head, by which we can relate to the world; and so on. A curious "septenary" argument was added in the second century A.D. by a Neo-Pythagorean philosopher of Arabia: the semen contributed by men during intercourse is ejaculated in seven spurts.[6]

A multiplicity of chambers or loculations in the uterus, like a multiplicity of wombs, would have important physiologic consequences. Aelian, a Roman writer (Claudius Adianus, A.D. 170-230), quoted Democritus as having established that the reason pigs and dogs bring forth many at birth is that they are provided with many receptacles for semen, since they have many wombs; and because the semen does not fill all at a single ejaculation, they find it necessary to copulate two, three, or more times, that the continuance of the act may properly fill the several receptacles. Aelian's hypothesis offered a scientific explanation for beastly lubricity.[7]

The human species, in contrast, had to contend only with the consequences of a double chamber. Semen falling on the right side would engender a male; if on the left, female offspring would result. What if both filled at the same time? Would unlike sexed twins be formed? The ancients did not tell us. Women desirous of having a son were advised to lie on the right side during and after coition. Up to the Renaissance, provident men who wished to control the sex of their offspring, followed the custom described by Aristotle (*Gen.Anim.* 765a, 23-5), which consisted in tying off in a bind the right or the left testicle during sexual intercourse, according as to whether they wished to procreate a girl or a boy, respectively.

The ancient Greeks also believed that the fetus fed inside the uterus, by sucking some of its flesh. The inner lining of the womb was thought to be provided with protuberances, one on each side, which resembled breasts, being broad at the base and tapering toward the tip. The wondrous design of Nature, many thought, had seen to it that the embryo acquire

early the habit of sucking at the maternal breast. No such
thing ever happens, corrected Aristotle (*Gen. Anim.* II, 7.
746a), since this has never been corroborated by dissections.
Moreover, the embryo is surrounded by membranes that
would impede its reaching such so-called protuberances. The
fetus is fed through the umbilical cord, the conduit that
brings it nutriment, and by no other route.

Soranus of Ephesus, one of the most learned and sagacious physicians of antiquity, who practised medicine in
Rome in the second century A.D., said the uterus has the
shape of a "cupping vessel" or "medicinal gourd." Its consistency he described as variable, the neck portion (cervix) feeling soft and fleshy in virgins, but tougher in women who had
given birth. He quoted Hierophilus, another medical authority who, with a knack for analogy that modern anatomists
and pathologists can appreciate, compared the consistency of
the virginal cervix to that of the tongue, and in women who
have borne children, to "the head of an octopus."[8] We are to
assume that the average ancient Greek was familiar with the
feel of the head of an octopus, otherwise the simile would
have seemed senseless.

That marine biology was very much a part of daily life
among the Greeks is also suggested by another stunning
anatomical concept. Diocles of Carystus, pioneer of dissection-
based anatomical studies who lived in the fourth century B.C.,
maintained that the uterus is provided with suckers, like
those on the tentacles of an octopus or a cuttlefish. We learn
this from the Stagirite (*Gen. Anim.* II, 7, 745b ff) who shared
this belief and was not alone in this regard, as suckers were
also mentioned by Hippocrates (*Aphorisms* V, 45) and others.

In Greek, the word for sucker, or cup-shaped hollow, is "cotyledon," a term that has survived in present-day anatomical terminology. It now designates a lobule of the placenta, composed of tufts of placental villi, whereas in ancient Greece it denoted the hypothetical uterine concavities into which the placenta was believed to insert.

These images of marine life have an obscure correspondence, one is tempted to say an arcane "sympathy," with life inside the womb. The fetus lives immersed in a liquid environment. In our earliest beginnings, we are all aquatic beings; and it is largely in this watery environment that we can best recognize ourselves as sons of Nature. For water is Mother: life-giving, eternal, fluid, unconstrained, infinitely spread. Life without it is impossible. Life started in the sea. It seems right that in our beginnings we be carried in a watery milieu, as if cradled in a soft embrace. Gaston Bachelard[9] remarked that of the four elements in Nature, only water is fit to form a cradle, and commented on a passage of Jules Michelet (1798-1874) that describes the primeval sea as "densely saturated by fatty atoms, adequate to the soft nature of the fish that lazily opens its mouth and ingests, thus being nourished *like an embryo in the bosom of the common mother*." (Italics added here for emphasis). The womb, by no coincidence, used to be called "the mother."

Moored by the umbilical cord, like fragile barks in an unfathomable sea, we rock to and fro, drifting on the tides of unthinking slumber as the gathering wind of life blows us toward an uncertain future. The sea is mother. A famous line of Homer calls Ocean the origin of all things (*Iliad* XIV, 246). Long before him, the pre-Socratics understood this, with

Thales the Milesian at the lead, who proclaimed water to be the original substance in the universe. But if the sea is mother, the converse is also true: the mother is sea. In the collective unconscious, life-giving Woman is identified with the sea. Marine shells, oysters and pearls are freighted with sexual symbolism. Mircea Eliade[10] reminds us that the bivalved shell bears a symbolic allusiveness that is directly gynecologic: its form suggests the external female genitals. The birth of Aphrodite from a shell is no gratuitous poetical fancy. It expresses the deep, obscure link between the goddess and the organic principle that constitutes the universal matrix, source and origination of everything that is.

Although the nature of Woman is wetness—*hygra physis*, as the Greeks put it—the watery milieu inside the womb is not entirely of maternal derivation. The amniotic fluid, of which the fetus is surrounded, is thought to come from many sources; however, as gestation advances, an increasing proportion of the total amount (800-1200 ml at term) is made of fetal urine. For a time, we may be said to swim in our own urine, although this excretion is very different from that formed in extrauterine life: in the womb, our inner ecology is still sterile, as yet uncontaminated by ingestions from the outer environment. And we swallow the fluid in which we are immersed, now and then taking drafts as a means for its disposal.

We also breathe it in. For a long time it was argued whether inspiratory movements take place before birth. A physiological activity on which our survival so strictly depends, could not be wholly untried before birth; some manner of "rehearsal" had to occur. This now appears to be so: the fetus makes vigorous inspiratory movements, some thirty percent of the time (periods without "breathing" may last more than one hour).[11] This draws fluid into the lungs, possibly enhancing the pulmonary development. Curiously, the lungs also secrete a fluid into the amniotic fluid, at the rate of 4 to 6 ml per kilogram of body weight per hour. Obstruction of the airway is known to result in too little amniotic fluid, and the liquid secretion damming up behind the level of the obstruction provokes overdistension of the lungs.[12]

The fetus, in conditions that decrease the volume of amniotic fluid, is a precious and fragile object bandied about woefully unprotected. Without the cushioning layer, the unborn are crowded inside the uterine cavity, and compacted by the walls of the womb. Infants thus constringed inside the maternal enclosure may be born in awkward postures, afflicted by orthopedic deformities. It is as if the still plastic tissues of a growing organism were placed in a narrow dungeon, the developing parts gradually squeezed by the unyielding walls. Thus the womb adds, to its unencumbered images, the sinister likeness of Inquisition torture chamber: a cruel device of progressively constricting walls.

One among the many prenatal perils results from too scanty an amount of amniotic fluid. I mean the presence of "amniotic bands," a term that is applied to remnants of membranes from the amniotic sac ("bag of waters") that take on a string-like or rope-like appearance and constrict the fetus. The constriction produces a deep encircling fissure, like that of a ring in a person whose hand swells inordinately while wearing it. Beyond the area of narrowing, the limb may be, if not wholly cut off, shriveled, atrophic, or variously deformed.

The origin of this accident is intriguing. A proposed mechanism envisions a very active fetus scratching the inner surface of the sac that encloses it. We imagine it digging with the nails, like a prisoner intent on escaping his dungeon with admirable patience and determination. The amniotic sac is multilayered, so that grating its inner surface, if the digging is not very deep, will not go through the entire thickness. Shreds or strips of amnion remain waving in the fluid, like algae in their marine habitat. These are called "Streeter's bands," in remembrance of the physician who described them.[13] The fetus moves its limbs haphazardly, and its limbs get caught in the waving strips, a process that is facilitated by the natural "stickiness" of the fetal tissues. The limb is caught usually by the fingers, which display the most active mobility. Further motioning will bring about greater entanglement, and the looping becomes tighter and tighter. The finger, the foot, the hand, or a whole leg, will be progressively constricted until it is made distorted, malconformed, or completely severed.

And Yet, It Moves . . .

Thus the uterus is not only protective lee, universal conveyance, avian image, watery enclosure, warm, maternal shelter and primitive abode, but also perilous space: a chamber set with traps that must be sorted before making an entrance in the world. It can constrict, but can it move? Few questions have been as hotly debated in medicine. There is little question that the uterus possesses some degree of mobility: it may be displaced en bloc in all directions, but to a very limited extent. Depending on the full or empty state of the rectum and the urinary bladder, it may rise or descend, or be flexed frontward or backward for a few millimeters. Lying on the flank displaces the uterine body ever so slightly to the corresponding side; lying on the genu-pectoral position (resting on knees and chest) straightens it to some extent. All these displacements, however, are extremely restricted. A number of vessels, fibrous bands, sheets of tissue (broad ligaments) and muscles fix the uterus in its normal anatomical position.

These facts could not have been ignored altogether by physicians in the past. Dissections and observations in cadavers of women dying from traumatic wounds were done in very ancient times. However, the concept of a uterus possessing autonomous mobility, manifesting violent displacements through the interior of the female body, and impinging upon other structures to cause a variety of diseases, was to prove uncommonly tenacious. The idea of a "wandering womb" therefore must have fulfilled an important cultural need of the societies in which it prospered.

Historians inform us that Egyptian documents written two thousand years before Christ, like the Kahun papyrus, ascribe many somatic complaints to abnormal encroachment of organs by a displaced womb;[14] and the Ebers papyrus (about 1500 B.C.) already mentions those remedies that classical Greco-Roman medicine propagated much later in the West. On the authority of several surviving works from classical antiquity, we know some of these remedies in detail.

The wayward uterus was attracted to its normal location by sitting the patient over a pail containing agreeable, perfumed solutions. The measures to repel it from an abnormal location were more drastic. The patient was made to inhale fetid, unpleasant odors, such as charred deer's horn, extinguished lamp wicks, squashed bedbugs, skins and rags, and all manner of substances with oppressive odors, which were sometimes anointed on the woman's nose and ears. Hippocrates introduced into the patient's vagina a small pipe, through which air was blown by means of a smithy's bellows. This measure was thought to correct the supposedly abnormal, twisted position of the uterus, by distending it. Others advocated the production of very loud noises, such as obtained from beating pans or metal plates, as an expedient to scare the mobile uterus back to its normal place. Sentience, in addition to spontaneous movement, seems to have been accepted as one of the faculties of the womb.

This concept, which today strikes us as absurd and incomprehensible, survived in some form until the nineteenth century; its residues until the twentieth, imbedded in the concept of "hysteria." This medical and psychiatric term only recently was deleted from the official terminology of contemporary human medicine.

In the third book of *Pantagruel*, Rabelais pokes fun at the idea of the wandering womb. He would not exempt the ministers of the healing arts from the scathing strokes of his pen, even though he was himself a full-fledged physician, a graduate of the renowned School of Medicine of Montpelier, medical Mecca in his time. In the mentioned work, a medico, Rondibilis, explains the reasons for the feminine character deficiencies. The chief one is organic and physiologic: women happen to harbor in their bodies an independent beast, the womb. "I call it an animal," says Rondibilis, "in accordance with the Academics as well as the Peripatetics. For if movement, as Aristotle says, is a sure sign of something animate, and if all that moves of itself is to be called an animal, then Plato was right when he called this thing an animal, having noted in it those movements commonly accompanying suffocation, precipitation, corrugation and indignation, movements sometimes so violent, that the woman is thereby deprived of all other senses and power of motion, as though she had suffered heart failure, syncope, epilepsy, apoplexy, or something very like death."[15]

The verbal exuberance, the piling up of synonyms and spinning off of adjectives, is pure Rabelais. The misogyny is typically medieval, in spite of the fact that Rabelais has been accredited both as an illustrious figure of the cultured Middle Ages, and as a fine product of the Renaissance, respectively by medievalists and Renaissance scholars, who each claimed the Rabelaisian oeuvre as their proper field of investigation (proof that Rabelais remains very much alive, Tomasi di Lampedusa once remarked, for who would ever dispute over a cadaver?).

The point is, the Western medical tradition accepted the concept of the womb as "animal within an animal," which had been transmitted from antiquity via the Hippocratic writings. And in this regard it is well to recall that, throughout the Middle Ages, Christian monks ensured the survival of ancient knowledge, including medical theories, by their sedulous copying of manuscripts. It is not difficult to imagine that the atmosphere in monastic houses, thick with irrational fears of sexuality and unbounded praise for celibacy and virginity, would not be favorable to women. The Aristotelian concept that woman represents a thwarted or incomplete man, a male *manqué*, was the official doctrine in medical teachings. By the same token, in religio-philosophical discourse, the biological inferiority of women was posited as one major cause of their dangerousness to men, and strengthened the conviction that women ought to conform to the demands of patriarchal society.

The low esteem of the womb did not end with the advent of the Renaissance. Thomas Willis (1621-1675), famous anatomist whose name is familiar to all physicians through its association with a ring of blood vessels at the base of the brain, emphatically asserted that it was impossible for the uterus to move, since it was "so strictly tied by neighboring structures round about" that it could not be displaced. The eminent Thomas Sydenham (1624-1689), justly regarded by some as the "father of internal medicine, " reiterated this view, but, like all physicians of his time, continued to speak of "hysterical passion," and thus to promote the idea that the womb was the cause of systemic manifestations, albeit through mechanisms unknown.

It seems that the concept of "hysteria" as a disease of the mind may be traced to Sydenham's work. However, as illustrious a man as Sir William Harvey, discoverer of the circulation of the blood in 1628, endorsed the belief in the wandering womb. In his monograph "On Parturition," he set down the unreserved affirmation that "grievous symptoms arise when the uterus either rises up or falls down."[16]

That valid, scientific knowledge and rational understanding are often insufficient to do away with erroneous belief, is a truism that the story of the wandering womb confirms. The uterus, many a medical man was persuaded, though it be so strongly attached that it cannot move, yet manages to roam about, as a writer of the period put it, "with petulant movements" that are "ascending, descending, convulsive, vagrant, prolapsed." The womb was believed to wreak havoc in the female organism by rising to the liver, spleen, diaphragm, stomach, breast, heart, lung, and as high as the throat or the head.

Why would the womb take to this obstinate, rebellious instability? What impelled the uterus to move about tumultuously and so disrupt the body's harmony? On this point medical opinion was unified. A womb-turned-mutineer hankered for male semen. Its riotous conduct was the result of unfulfillment. As long as it would be kept away from its proper function, which is procreation, it would fall prey to the frenzied distemper that was the root cause of hysteria and its multiple manifestations.

Accordingly, official medicine advised early marriage and closely spaced pregnancies; for only by keeping the "animal within an animal" constantly satiated, would its fits and spasms be avoided. Mind you, there was no question of disobeying the dictates of conventional morality. No one recommended free sex. The honor of maidens had to be preserved. Chastity was valued in society and extolled by religion. Decorum and propriety enjoined a modest behavior in widows. But, barring formal interdiction from customs or religion, it was best to keep the beast satiated. It was a matter of sound prophylaxis.

Dutch painters in the seventeenth and eighteenth centuries reveled in the realistic depiction of innumerable scenes of domestic life. There is perhaps no richer iconographic record of women afflicted with *hysterica passio, furor uterinus,* hysteria, or whichever name was used to designate illness thought to result from the restlessness of a wayward womb.

Jan Steen, Dirck Hals, Jacob Ostervelt, Franz van Mieris, and many other Dutch painters tried their hand at representing the theme of the "sick maiden," that is, a young woman repining at home, weary and wan, attended by relatives or visited by a physician, and suffering from what, in the context of historical knowledge, may properly be interpreted as hysteria, also known as "suffocation of the mother."

In several paintings by Jan Steen (1626-1679), a languishing, pale girl is examined by a physician. At least eighteen versions of the medical examination theme were executed by this meticulous recorder of scenes of daily life. "The Doctor's Visit" is the title given to an easel exhibited at the Wellington Museum, Apsley House, London. In this painting, the diagnosis is not in doubt: the patient is a lovesick girl. The allusions from which this inference may be drawn are patent: a little boy, on the left lower corner of the painting, plays with arrows that he aims, like a young Cupid, at the viewer. A large canvas, suspended on the back wall, represents an amorous scene of the story of Venus and Adonis.

In another "Doctor's Visit" from Steen's brush, this one kept at the Philadelphia Museum of Art, the doctor is taking a sick girl's pulse, while several personages engage in merry activities, such as music playing, buffoonery, and joke telling, presumably to combat her melancholy. Still another rendering of the same theme, exhibited in the Taft Museum of Cincinnati, Ohio, depicts a young woman who reclines as if swooning, while an unprepossessing, unfashionably attired physician (a quack?) bends toward her to take her pulse, and a matron—either the girl's mother or, more likely, a maid—watches the proceedings. Again, there is little question of the etiology of the disease: in the background, on the right, the obligatory canvas with a mythologic, erotic scene; and on the foreground, on the left, an open book with an inscription stating that against the ravages of love no medicine avails.

Common to these and other paintings of the period, is a curious detail. Somewhere on the floor of the sickroom, the attentive viewer will discover a length of ribbon close to, or trailing into, a charcoal burner. The latter was a household item commonly encountered in Holland, and used as a warming device in Northern latitudes. The use of the ribbon, however, was less obvious, and elicited some discussion among scholars.[17] In some paintings, an attendant is holding a ribbon, or a secondary personage appears to be bringing it into the room. It is now clear that this was a therapeutic adjunct. The acrid smoke of a burning ribbon was thought to be helpful in bringing back the patient from a swoon, or restoring the spirits of those sunk in torpor or enfeebled by lassitude.

Doctor Thomas Sydenham recommended to bring a burning blue ribband under a patient's nose as a means to combat the languor of the women afflicted with hysterical symptoms. Clearly, this measure was not invented trusting solely in the restorative powers of strong smells. We may not be conscious of it, but the popular custom of using smelling salts, ammonia, camphor, or other strong odoriferous compounds to alleviate states of lethargy, languor, and fainting, traces its origin directly to the ancient attribution of waywardness and obduracy to the womb. Strong odors were thought to chase a displaced uterus away from abnormal locations.

In our time, discussions on uterine mobility have ceased. A chastened womb seems quietly to occupy its undistinguished pelvic seat, like any other viscus. The trouble is, the womb is not like any other viscus. Its place in men's imagination still looms large, and it continues to evoke emotions that range from awe and reverential fascination, to outright fear and ill disguised hostility. Male surgeons remove twice as many uteri as female surgeons.[18] Feminists have complained that no organ has suffered from so much surgical aggression, or been removed upon pretexts as flimsy, as the human uterus.

Nor is femaleness the sole factor determining its vulnerability to the unscrupulous surgical scalpel. A survey in Switzerland showed that the lifetime prevalence of hysterectomy was 29.9 percent among the less well educated, compared to only 12.9 percent among highly educated women.[19] "Perhaps fortunately for male patients, " wryly commented the surveyors, "no female urologists practiced on the Swiss health market scene."

Similarly, investigators in Baltimore concluded that black women were more than twice as likely to have a diagnosis of uterine "fibroids" (the tumors that are the main reason for performing a hysterectomy) as white women; blacks were also more likely to have complications, longer hospitalization, and three times the in-hospital mortality rate of whites.[20] Thus, of approximately 600,000 hysterectomies performed annually in the United States,[21] it seems that many are suspect, that is, carried out for reasons other than legitimate medical indication.

Is it surprising that an organ that has been, among other things, gourd, bottle, jug, suction cup, wineskin, cradle, bird, octopus, primeval sea, and animal-within-an-animal, should adopt yet one more guise? It now becomes mirror held up to our society. And it is not its fault if the reflection is uncomely.

On Female "Impressionism"

The Ease of Imprinting

FOR ALL THAT THE FEMALE GERM IS MASSIVE, SLOW, AND languorous, its sensitivity to stimuli is extreme. Let a single, tiny sperm cell, one among millions vying for access, penetrate its substance, and a prodigious cascade of phenomena will be triggered: an incredibly complex series of ill understood changes that results in a new human being. There seems to be a disproportion here, a lack of correspondence between the apparent minuteness or triviality of the cause, and the overwhelming complexity of the effect. Little wonder that for a long time the best minds uniformly believed that the cause could not reside in what they saw. There had to be a transcendent, immaterial, unperceived mechanism. Something that escaped detection by our senses, these being too coarse for the subtleness of such agency. This is why it was felt that a mere vapor, an invisible, mysterious efflux ascending from the male secretion, communicated its procreative powers to the female cell. This was all that was required to irritate the egg-cell into beginning the formation of a new being.

This idea thrived in the brain of the best researchers, including Lazzaro Spallanzani (1729-1799), the Italian savant who steered research on reproduction toward a trustworthy experimental path. He was the first to demonstrate that actual physical contact between male and female germs is the *sine qua non* condition for fertilization to occur. [1]

Schoolboys are not known to relish dry studies on the history of science. But, as Pinto-Correia says humorously in her lively and engrossing book, *The Ovary of Eve*,[2] they are apt to remember that abbot Spallanzani was the man who fitted frogs with boxer shorts. Indeed, this impressive man, this staid scientist and learned scholar, (who eventually was ordained into the Catholic Church), did just that.

His observations had led him to hypothesize that the action of semen upon the female egg was not exerted at a distance, much in spite of received ideas then current. The force of universal gravitation and its laws had just been explained by the genial Mr. Newton. As happens any time that a momentous discovery takes place, investigators in every field of enquiry were anxious to apply the novel universal principle to their own unsolved problems. The most orthodox and widespread persuasion among biologists was that gravitation had a role in animal fertilization. Or, if not gravity, a form of energy akin to it, invisible and immaterial, some kind of "animal electric fluid," often referred to as *aura seminalis,* which had the ability to rise from semen, reach the ovum, and penetrate it (perhaps through tiny "pores" on its surface) in order to spark off the complex process of gestation. Not so, protested Spallanzani. If a barrier is interposed between the male's ejaculate and the female's egg, conception cannot take place.

Let the barrier be ever so tenuous, so long as it is impermeable to semen it will effectively preclude fertilization. And here was the grave, solemn, imposing man of learning, cutting away and sewing up little breeches in taffeta, muslin, or calico, with which he dressed up his male frogs. Those so attired could not engender offspring. No matter how many times they embraced the female, or how passionately; their ardor was sterile, because the ejaculate was stopped by the garment. Remove the underwear, and the fertilizing potency of these same male frogs was restored.

In no way did this mean that the male influence was coarsely material. Its airy nature could not be doubted, particularly in view of the results of Spallanzani's subsequent experiments. He took two concave glass dishes and placed them one on top of the other. The top one contained frog eggs, the lower one frog semen. No tadpole ever developed, and these negative results were again observed when the position of the dishes was reversed, *i.e.*, semen on top, eggs below. No fertilization took place even when Spallanzani sealed with wax the edges of the sperm-containing dish, in order to avoid the possible evaporation and dispersion of the invisible *aura seminalis*. At length, the evidence was compelling: the action of semen is by direct contact, not mediated by an unperceived "fluid" or *aura seminalis*. But the nature of this action was still of such an order as might be called insubstantial or ethereal in more than one respect. Consider our man's further work.

Spallanzani mixes sperm with water: three grains of seed in one pound of water (1 pound = 489 grams = 16 ounces; 1 ounce = 576 grains). This mixture is effective: fertilization takes place. Then he uses a higher dilution: eighteen ounces of water; the results again are positive. Then, he contrives a further refinement: he places 5 grains of frog sperm in 18 ounces of water, and he sinks a needle in this preparation. With the same needle, he touches the surface of frog eggs. Marvel of marvels, the result is fecundation. As he put it, "spermatized water" is effective. And, since he feels comfortable with mathematics, he sits down to perform some calculations, from which he arrives at the following interesting conclusions:

The volume of the frog's egg, relative to the volume of seed that is necessary to fertilize it, is as 1,064,777,777 is to 1. The volume of the male seed is 1 / 3,002,120,420 of a cubic line ("line" being an old, now disused unit of length measurement equivalent to 1 /12 inch). And the weight of the male seed is 1 / 2,994,687,500 of a grain.

In other words, an infinitesimal amount of male seed is all that is needed to impregnate the female. The female germ had to be extraordinarily susceptible to the male's influence, but the male germ, in its turn, gave evidence of a formidable power. Need one say that this incredible potency suggested an uncommon, extremely subtle form of energy, bordering on the preternatural?

Spallanzani never attributed any major importance to spermatozoa. Sure, the restless "animalcules" were present, always moving about spasmodically, in semen. They had been observed by a growing number of investigators since microscopy became available, namely for at least a hundred years before Spallanzani's experiments. But their role in reproduction did not seem credible. Not to Spallanzani, anyway. For it did violence to common sense to propose that those tadpole-like, erratic creatures should have anything to do with the generation of an organized animal of a higher order, let alone the noblest being in all Creation, man. To the end, the good abbot continued to believe that spermatozoa were contaminants, living forms that, in any case, were utterly unimportant for human reproduction.

What seized the imagination irresistibly, was the strength of "spermatized water." It could only be compared to the most toxic poisons known to mankind, like those of venomous snakes, of which a few drops can fell a brawny giant. What could be the nature of the energy that had been communicated to the water by the male seed? It brought to mind that other recently discovered, formidable natural energy, electricity, whose actions in the body were being studied around that time by the likes of Luigi Galvani (1737-1798) and Alessandro Volta (1745-1827). Was it not true that in a dramatic public demonstration the jaw of a recently executed criminal was seen to contract, and the extended fingers of one of his hands flex into a fist, thanks to the uncanny virtues of this "fluid"? If electricity could reactivate the parts of a dead body, surely it could be the agent that prompted the fertilized egg into the series of processes that characterize gestation.

That this idea persisted, albeit in modified form, down to the nineteenth century, may seem incredible. It is nonetheless in evidence in a work of a prominent physician, Carl Friedrich Burdach, whose name may be familiar to many students of neuroanatomy (a nerve tract in the posterior spinal cord, or *fasciculus cuneatus,* is sometimes referred to as Burdach's fascicle). No longer did he speak of aura seminalis, the turn was now of electricity. Sexual attraction between man and woman he compared to the static electricity between two poles of different sign, which incites a chemical reaction of synthesis.

The attraction grows progressively with proximity, "just as tension grows between two electrical bodies animated of contrary polarities when they are mutually approximated without being able to discharge themselves." And just as the electrical current is instantaneously spread out in conducting media, so the lovers feel the jolt of their passion, and "an electrical conflict is manifested in the power of the gaze of the two beings fettered by the chains of love." More to the point, "the woman who has conceived describes what she experienced as an electrical discharge."[3]

On the other hand, regardless of the nature of the male prolific energy, not much of it was needed, given the female seed's exquisite sensitivity to external stimuli. A little thing could set it going; a simple breeze sufficed. Indeed, it is a belief of very ancient roots that the breeze could impregnate. In ancient Greek poetry, the wind, in various personifications (Boreas, Zephyr) was supposed to have had fertile carnal union with nymphs. But perhaps the most famous of those assertions is the attribution of the same power to the unpersonified wind by the Roman poet Virgil (Publius Vergilius Maro: B.C. 70-19). He wrote in his *Georgics* that mares, when ready to mate, especially in the spring, ". . . when heat returns to the bones, stand atop cliffs with their mouths open toward the zephyr, and they inhale the gentle breeze; and often, without copulation—marvelous to tell—impregnated by the wind they scatter among the rocks, and valleys and ravines . . ." (Bk. III, 270-276).[4]

Such a story was repeated by a number of ancient authors. It could not have passed unnoticed by Pliny the Elder (A.D. 23-79), the greatest compiler of lies and fantastic stories who ever lived, and who imputed this reproductive method to the mares that live on the banks of the Tagus river in Lusitania (present-day Portugal). These quadrupeds, says Pliny in his *Natural History*, as soon as they feel a west wind blowing, stand facing it and thus they become pregnant. However, the foal produced by this means does not live above three years (whereas our author gives fifty years as the limit of a horse's longevity. Stallions, he points out, go on serving to the age of thirty-three, and a stallion was reported to have continued his "service" to forty, but then "he needed assistance in lifting his forequarters").[5]

Birds were also thought to conceive without copulation. The idea dates back at least to Aristotle, who in his treatise on *The Generation of Animals* (book III, 749b) set it down that in some birds embryos are formed spontaneously, and that these are called "wind-eggs" or "zephyria." The reason given by the Stagirite is that birds do not menstruate, so that much residual (generative) "matter" accumulates in them. Recall that, for this philosopher, during reproduction the female contributes "matter" and the male furnishes "form." Birds not much given to flight, like hens, or those with proportionately large bodies, like pigeons, are likely to hoard matter in excess. This is in contrast with active birds and birds of prey, like falcons, in whom the said matter is derived to the formation of large feathers and strong wings, whereas the body remains relatively small, hot, and dry; such birds, in consequence, do not lay many eggs. For "what Nature takes from one place is added to the other."[6]

Another Roman writer, Aelian (Claudius Aelianus: born *circa* 170 A.D.) repeated the notion that all vultures are female. These birds, fearing childlessness, fly against the east wind and open their beaks to it, by which means they are impregnated as they receive the onrush of wind into the throat. Aelian extended the prolific virtue of the wind to sheep, to whom he attributed conscious knowledge of this property. For he assured us that sheep, being aware that the north wind produces males and the south wind females, know very well what to do: a sheep that is being covered faces in one direction or the other, according to the sex of the offspring that it desires. Shepherds share this knowledge, and put the rams to the sheep when the south wind is blowing, so as to ensure that their offspring be preferably female.[7]

As might be expected, the alleged ability to conceive unassisted that is displayed by sheep, mares and birds, was made extensive to the female of the human species. A rich fantastic literature, whose origin scholars trace to ancient China, made reference to mythical countries inhabited exclusively by women. Dispensing with males, they were impregnated by inanimate objects, such as the wind, fruits of a tree that they ingested, or certain waters.

In other versions of this legend, they would mate with men kept as slaves for the sole purpose of reproduction, or with men that, like lost sailors and explorers, now and then accidentally stumbled into their domain. Some stories depict the women of these lands as breeding only females, others as being delivered of both, male and female infants, but regularly disposed to commit infanticide with the former and raise only the latter.

The Chinese stories made reference to three countries inhabited exclusively by women. One was in the Far West, called Fu-lin, and scholars believe it may have corresponded to the Eastern Roman Empire. A second country of women, said to lie to the south, is tentatively identified with a region of India inhabited by tribes that practiced polyandry. The third country, purely mythical, stood somewhere in the China sea. The various stories of the Chinese lore passed on to the Middle East, there to be retold with the fantastic embellishments for which Arabian literature is justly famous.[8]

In the West, wind-impregnation of women came by and by to be talked about as a joke. By the time of the Renaissance, the general feeling was that voiced by Pierre Bourdeille, better known as abbot Brantôme (1540-1614), celebrated ribald story teller of the Renaissance. Brantôme claimed, in the second "discourse" of his *Lives of Gallant Ladies*, that many husbands "would rather have their wives find such a wind as might make them feel less hot, without going to look for their lovers, there to fit on their spouses' heads an ugly pair of horns." But, joking aside, the idea that Woman could conceive with no other help than that provided by the wind, continued to have some advocates. Chief among the later ones was Claude Perrault (1613-1688), brother of Charles, the author of universally well known fairy tales for children ("Little Red Riding Hood,"and "Puss in Boots," among others).

Claude was not only a physician-naturalist, but also an architecture *aficionado*. Despite the lack of appropriate credentials, his influential brother got him appointed as an architect in the works of renovation of the Louvre. Here, he collaborated together with three famous architects in the design of the magnificent east facade of this palace, with its majestic Colonnade. This was probably his foremost achievement, since he left no permanent mark in the biological sciences.

In his dissertation of 1676 (*Mémoire pour servir à l'histoire des animaux, ou traité sur la méchanique des animaux*), he defends the old idea of "panspermia," the notion that germs or rudimentary forms of life exist in the air, which, under appropriate conditions, may be turned into active form. It exceeded his understanding, as it baffled the most eminent intellectuals of his time (and, we might add, of two centuries to come), that a highly differentiated, supremely well organized living being, with numerous and varied structures, could come out of a liquid (*i.e*, the seminal fluid and/or the female secretions) no matter how elaborately compounded, fermented, decanted, or distilled. It was simpler, and appeared to place much less strain on credibility, to imagine the presence of tiny, invisible beings, already formed but still not animated.

These preformed living entities—named "organic molecules," "germs,"and so on—awaited incorporation into the proper milieu to unfold in all their splendor. Certainly, these "germs" could develop in the body of a woman without any need for male intervention. But, in general, a man's participation was preferable, because the unique qualities of the *aura seminalis* made the male ejaculate the fittest medium for growth and development of the "germ."

The historian Pierre Darmon tells us, in his engrossing *History of Procreation in the Age of the Baroque*[9], that on the 13th day of January of 1637, the Parliament of Grenoble exonerated from all guilt a woman, named Magdelaine d'Aumont d'Aiguemère, accused of adulterous relationships, who gave birth to an infant after her husband had been away uninterruptedly for several years. Female impressionability was a factor that learned jurists considered relevant in arriving to the verdict.

The lady had thought with rare intensity of her absent spouse, and had a dream in which she represented his image most vividly. This yearning must have contributed to prepare her body to receive the seed. The hypertrophic sensitivity of the female soul, when stirred by such wistful reveries, desires and reminiscences, is apt to cause bodily changes favorable to the inception of pregnancy. But, of course, by themselves, these emotions may not have been enough. However, it so happened that during that dream she left the window of her bedroom open. She tossed and turned in bed, agitated by her dream. The sheets were in disarray, and her sleeping gown was raised to close to the level of her waist. And the "organic molecules," "vermicular germs," "worm-like rudiments," or whichever name the advocates of panspermia chose to designate the floating, inchoate embryos that existed in the air, found a way to insinuate themselves into the bedroom, then via the exposed genitalia of the sleeping woman, straight through, to her womb.

This interpretation was not arrived at by primitive people in thrall to ignorance and superstition, or living in a remote place barred from all enlightenment, but by high officers of a civilized European country, in an urban site, and at a time when major contributions to the arts and sciences were being made by many of their compatriots. On the same year that the Parliament of Grenoble officially sanctioned the occurrence of an instance of wind-impregnation, Descartes published his

Discourse of the Method, having already published other important works. Which is why we are inclined to readily assent to Darmon's contention, based on some documentary evidence, that behind it all there must have been a sordid tale of politics and family feuding. The relatives of the absent husband must have been troubled at the thought that an undeserving wife appeared ready to grab a major share of the family fortune, and the lady must have been eager to legitimize a baby that had descended upon her "out of the blue sky," or, as her defensors might have said, from its airy abode, at a most inopportune juncture.

It must also be recalled that the ideas underlying the so-called "panspermia" are ancient indeed. The first formulation antedates Vergil and the other Greco-Roman writers that spoke of the impregnation of birds and Andalousian mares by gusts of wind or jets of water. The roots of this belief can be traced at least as far back as the pre-Socratic thinkers.

Heraclitus of Ephesus (*c.*540-*c.*480 B.C.) taught that the principle of the universe, the creative energy from which the world originated, and which he identified with a mixture of fire and water, existed dispersed in all things, including the air that we breathe. Therefore, with each inhalation we inspire some of this vital principle, which was also the principle of biological development. Whether he meant that material particles capable of originating new life are suspended in the air, or whether this is abusive exegesis, is best left to the experts to discuss. Not in vain did his contemporaries nickname him "the Obscure."

Except for fragments, no work of Heraclitus exists. This is true of all the initiators of Greek philosophy. Recall that what the pre-Socratic philosophers said is known mostly through the few fragments that survived the ravages of time, or through quotations from later writers, who repeated their predecessors' statements mainly in order to refute them. And this gives us a measure of the ancient thinkers' stature; for as Bertrand Russell once pointed out, they must have been pretty good, since even when quoted by their opponents they still manage to look great. Imagine what the majority of present-day intellectuals would look like, if we knew them only through recollections sifted by the malice of their enemies!

Truly it may be asserted, as did Diderot in his celebrated conversation with D'Alambert, that the female egg-cell "topples all the schools of theology and all the temples of the earth." For the ovocyte is nothing but an insentient mass, a highly complex aggregate of inert materials—and today's scientists agree that it is no more than a living cell, which they define as an aggregate of macromolecules in extremely complex but definable dynamic equilibrium—in which the male seed is introduced. But the male seed itself is an assemblage of macromolecules in complicated equilibrium. And "with an inert matter, arranged in a certain way, impregnated with another inert matter, plus heat and movement, we obtain sensibility, life, memory, consciousness, passions, thought . . ."[10]

That out of the female seed, a microscopic corpuscle measuring about 100 μ in diameter, should develop a whole human being with its myriad constituents, continues to be one of the knottiest problems, if not *the* central mystery, for biology.

Modern investigators have corroborated the ancient belief that a minimal stimulus can launch the expression of the astounding potential locked in the female seed; but they have been more concerned with defining the specific ways in which this happens. Jacques Loeb (1859-1924), of the Rockefeller Research Institute, working with sea-urchins in the marine biology laboratory of Woods Hole, Massachusetts, established that the unfertilized egg may be made to divide (parthenogenesis), resulting in the production of normal larvae, by exposure to defined chemicals. The message to divide, Loeb established, is chemical. Which gave occasion to a facetious French scientist, today largely forgotten, to refer to Loeb's experimental subjects as "those little citizens, the sons of Mrs. Urchin and Mr. Magnesium Chloride."

It is one thing to induce parthenogenetic divisions in the eggs of frogs, newts, or sea urchins. It is another, of a very different order of magnitude, to obtain the like results in mammals. Hence the sensational nature of the announcement in 1977 by Karl Illmensee, a German professor working at the university of Geneva, and Peter Hoppe, his collaborator from Bar Harbor, Maine, that they had been able to produce "uniparental" mice.[11] These investigators reported successful experiments in which the ovocytes of mice were divested of their nuclei, and replaced with nuclei taken from cells of early mouse embryos. Thus outfitted, the ovocytes went on to divide. After short term culture in the laboratory, the embryos were implanted in a carrier mother. The mice produced in this fashion (*i.e.*, in spite of never having had the benefit of male seed, . . . not even a whiff of *aura seminalis*!) were, of course, clones of the embryos that donated the replacement nuclei:— the episode belongs in the history of cloning.

Unfortunately, no one could reproduce these experiments.

The operation was apparently a model of micromanipulative dexterity: the ovocyte's nuclear extirpation, and the introduction of the replacement nucleus, were reportedly carried out in a single stage, thus reducing the trauma to the egg-cell to a single microinjection. The problem was, the ablest, most dexterous micromanipulators, and the most minutious laboratory workers, were consistently foiled; for when the nuclear transfer was accomplished, the egg-cell did not progress beyond a few divisions before dying. At length, the universal failure cast an aura of suspicion upon the researchers. An investigative commission was appointed; and although no wrongdoing or willful misrepresentation was ever demonstrated, the work of these investigators came to an end amidst unseemly rumors.

Two other investigators in this same field, Davor Solter and James McGrath, finally decided to publish their negative results in 1984, peremptorily announcing that parthenogenesis in mammals is biologically impossible.[12] (Later, the success in cloning proved them wrong). It is not customary among top scientists to publish negative results, nor are such communications received with alacrity by the editors of the most prestigious journals in the scientific community. However, in this case, together with the declaration of bafflement came an explanation of its cause, and, as it turned out, the opening up of an important new chapter in molecular genetics.

It became clear that, in mammals, the process of *gametogenesis*, i.e., the maturation of the male and female germ-cells (ovocytes or spermatozoa), is accompanied by changes in the DNA of certain genes. These modifications are such that the genes concerned are "silenced," that is, they are rendered inactive. This phenomenon is now known as "genetic imprinting."

The paternal and maternal genes are different, and both are present in normal cells. But since one or the other may be put out of commission in maturing germ-cells, it seems that both must be present in the developing embryo, in order to compensate for the loss due to genetic imprinting.

Maternal Impressions

Science tries to define how the female seed responds to the inciting stimuli of procreation. But the common notion has long been afoot, that sensitivity and sensibility are fundamental feminine attributes. Not mere accidents of the germ-cell, but radical peculiarities of Woman. If, as the Aristotelian school of thought maintained, Woman furnishes the "matter" in generation, and man the "form," it is because she was identified as the source of all that is ductile, plastic, or malleable: the clay to which man, the potter, can impart a shape. She is pliable: her disposition is uniquely capable of taking in impressions from outside. She is receptive: apt to incorporate the influences of the external environment, like a metal that, under the influence of the lodestone, becomes itself magnetized. Now, the imagination was often compared to a very powerful magnet, one whose radius of action was quite vast, so that it could activate or bedevil every area of the mind. It could scramble, confuse and disarrange thoughts and emotions. Women, by their very nature, were prone to such distemper. Wrote Vandermonde, an eighteenth century physician:

> "Physicians know that the bodies that give low-pitched sounds vibrate more slowly than those whence we draw high-pitched sounds. Thus, the more a string is tensed, the

more acutely it will express the impression that it has received. We know very well that the strings of Woman are more delicate and finer than those of Man, therefore more sensitive; the exterior objects act upon their senses with greater force; they are represented with greater liveliness, and the passions that result therefrom are stronger. Women are more subject to love and to inconstancy; this is a natural consequence of their structure [. . .] Their fibers are fitter to be affected by the objects that irritate their sensibility, because their tension is stronger, and the vibrations faster; but the easing is more considerable as well. The relaxation follows the former state of constraint, and because their fibers are weaker, they have more trouble in regaining the tension. There remains therefore a despondency that hampers the soul's desire and produces disgust and inconstancy. When women are restrained by reason and duty, more is their honor and greater their merit, since they have greater difficulty to master themselves . . ."[13]

Could this high receptivity fail to affect the fetus? It is a fact that what we see in others exerts an effect on the corresponding part of our own body. Thus, seeing a person with an unsightly blemish or an ulcer in a limb, will provoke a strange sensation, an itching or a horripilation in the same site of the limb of the observer. Descartes explained that this is because the "animal spirits" (*esprits animaux*), as Descartes originally called what today may be rendered as "nervous impulses," are directed toward that bodily part. In the case of a pregnant woman, these animal spirits—which Descartes and his followers imagined as some kind of vaporous factors traveling in the blood stream—would not only localize in her own body, but would also be derived toward the fetal body, always at the same or corresponding part.

Hence the prophylactic measure devised by early Cartesian philosophers, that if a mother happens to watch an unsightly spectacle with potential bodily impact, say a person being wounded on a leg, it is recommended that she rub vigorously some other bodily part, or tickle it, on the assumption that this maneuver will send some animal spirits on a detour, and impede their excessive concentration in the part at risk.

Nicolas Malebranche (1638-1715), French theologian and philosopher who championed his own brand of Cartesianism, tells us in his "Search of Truth"[14] that about nine years before setting down to compose this major work, he had known a young man, an inmate at an institution for patients beyond the pale of medical science, the *Hôpital des Incurables*, who had been born mad, and whose body appeared, since birth, broken in various sites. The man lived to his twenties, and a noteworthy observation was that the places of his body that were "broken" (presumably deformed by skeletal fractures or bends) corresponded to the places upon which torture was usually applied to convicted criminals, as decreed by the barbarous laws prevailing in those times. According to the principles that the philosopher had established, this unfortunate birth could be explained as a consequence of the mother having witnessed, while pregnant, the torture administered to a criminal. For then every blow dealt to the criminal had hit with great force the imagination of the mother, and by a kind of contrecoup, the shock had been transmitted to the delicate and tender brain and body of her child.

Moreover, proceeds the philosopher's argumentation, while still fetuses in their mothers' wombs, the future children are in a state of profound feebleness and extreme privation, which determines the very close union they must maintain with their mothers in order to live. And their bodies being so closely joined to the maternal organism, it is only natural that they should have the same sentiments, and the same passions, as the mother. They see what she sees (this, under present concepts, is not possible), and hear what she hears (in this, Malebranche was, in the main, correct).

Consider how the vivid facial expressions of a man are able to inspire a like sentiment in those who see him at close range, even if they are not related to him. How more likely, then, that the same sentiments that agitate a mother be passed on to the child she harbors in her womb. For the fetal and maternal bodies are joined as one: blood and animal spirits are shared in common by these two. And since the emotions and sentiments are but the natural consequence of movements and changes in the animal spirits, it stands to reason that the movements of these spirits should be communicated from the mother to the child.

It is still necessary to add that the effects of these changes are not the same for everyone. Hardened soldiers are not moved by the sight of a massacre; executioners will not stop their deadly tasks out of feelings of compassion. Women and children, however, are naturally compassionate. They suffer grievously from seeing others suffer. Forceful movements of animal spirits must produce in them serious effects. Fragility, delicacy of structure and liability of sentiment, are, in this scheme, the fundamental characteristics accounting for damage. Woman is impressionable, but the unborn is still more so.

These considerations help to explain why the spectacle of a man put to the torture, when watched by the pregnant woman, caused congenital anomalies in her son. At the sight of the frightful execution, the violent agitation of the animal spirits traveled speedily toward the different parts of her body, and the corresponding parts of her child's body. But because the mother's skeleton was relatively strong, she experienced no ill effect. The fetal structures, being much weaker, could not resist the shock of the torrent of animal spirits released by the frightful sight. This is why her son came to the world destitute of reason and broken in various parts of his body. A tragedy that could have been averted, observes Malebranche with astounding self-assurance, by the simple expedient of rubbing or tickling the maternal body at some site. This would have deviated the animal spirits away from the bodily parts that were injured in her child.

Malebranche produces yet another personally observed instance. Fresh in his memory, for not more than one year had passed, says the philosopher, was the case of a Parisian woman who was a fervent votary of Saint Pius. She gazed with great devotion at the image of this saint during the festivities of his canonization, and in consequence of her great fervor, delivered an infant that was the splitting image of Saint Pius. The face of the newborn child was like the visage of an elderly man, looking as old as it is possible for an infant who lacks a beard. His arms were crossed on top of his chest, his eyes were raised toward the sky, and he had scarcely any forehead, because the image of this saint, "being placed on an elevation toward the vault of the church, and his visage being turned up toward heaven, presented, it too, very little forehead. It had a kind of overturned miter on the shoulders, with several rounded marks at the places where the miters are covered with gems. In sum, this child resembled very much the painting, after which his mother had formed him by the force of her imagination. This is something that all of Paris was able see, because [the child's body] was preserved in wine spirits for a long time."[15]

A striking example of the power of the imagination, not so much the mother's, as that of Nicolas Malebranche. The infant that he described so vividly resembled babies with *iniencephaly*, one of a group of complex congenital malformation of extreme severity, incompatible with more than fleeting extrauterine life. The unfortunate newborns so affected have a short neck associated with deficient growth of the cervical spine, in consequence of which the face appears directed upwards ("toward heaven"). Growth of the skull is markedly deficient, for this profound impairment is related to anencephaly. Because development of the brain and of the bones conforming the top of the skull is rudimentary, the forehead is markedly narrowed. In this, Malebranche saw an effect of the foreshortening of the saint's forehead in the portrait that the mother, to her misfortune, had watched too keenly; and the illusion of contraction was still enhanced by the elevated position of the painting.

In a closely related malformation, *exencephalus acrania*, the top of the skull does not develop, and the brain actually

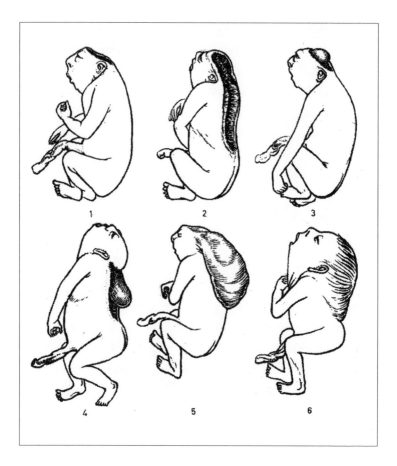

Anencephaly and other related malformations. These are serious malformations, and afflicted infants do not survive more than a few hours outside the maternal womb. On he lower row, large redundant sacs are present on the dorsum of the infant, which may contain ill-preserved brain substance. The dorsal sac suggested a monk's cowl to early observers. Note that, because of shortened, fused vertebrae of the neck, the afflicted infants appear to be looking upward.

(*From Morison, 1963*)

oozes out of the cranial cavity, coming to occupy an anomalous position under the skin, behind the head. This forms a pouch-like structure covered by the skin of the nape, which contains the poorly formed, gelatinous brain.[16] In this most grievous developmental aberration, Malebranche saw an overturned bishop's miter ornamented with jewels.

The fanciful correlations are endless. Jacques Blondel,[17] eighteenth century physician, quotes an episode that Jan Swammerdam (1637-1680), the famous Dutch microscopist, recorded in his book *Uteri mullieris Fabrica*. A woman of Utrecht was scared by the view of a black man. To preserve the whiteness of the child she was carrying, she washed herself head to toe. In due time, she delivered an infant that was white all over, except in places that she could not wash well enough (probably pigmented birthmarks), which retained some blackness.

A physician of Frankfurt reported that the wife of a casket maker, affrighted by the sight of a butcher who disemboweled a pig, gave birth to a son whose entrails were hanging out of the abdomen (well known defect of closure of the abdominal wall, known in medicine as *gastroschisis*). It is easy to understand how a pregnant woman, who rested under a cherry tree when suddenly startled by cherries falling on her lap, relates this experience to the fact that her newborn child presents cherry-red blotches on its skin (hemangiomas). But, Blondel explains, imagination may exert the direst effects on the psyche, not the body.

Indeed, the power of the imagination on mood and emotion cannot be denied. To hear his doctor formulate a good prognosis works wonders for a patient. A good surprise,

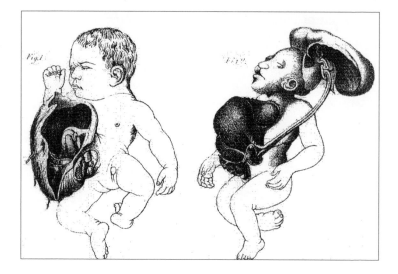

Congenital defects of closure of the body wall, with the extrusion of internal organs to the outside. This kind of congenital malformation, well known to specialists in neonatal diseases, led in the past to the popular belief that sensitive mothers who watched the eviscerations of animals could give birth to infants so afflicted.

(*From Geoffroy St. Hillaire*)

happy prospects, are undisputably beneficial in a physical sense. And the opposite is no less true: severe worries, unmitigated sorrows and cares can render a man frenetic, mad, or reduce him to imbecility. Violent passions have been known to trigger convulsions, chest pains, even sudden death: a criminal on the block has expired before the hatchet descended on his neck.

It could scarcely be doubted that commotions of such magnitude impact on the fetus. But what is the timing of their action? When can maternal impressions be transmitted to the fetus to leave their mark thereon? Is it during carnal union, at the very moment of conception? The latter proposition was considered by the experts only to deny it. For at that happy moment, in the heat of the embrace, the fancy is fully occupied and has no time to represent to itself disagreeable or repugnant objects. Monstrous, deformed, or character-deficient babies are not fashioned this way. Nothing farther away from imagination at that time, than the thought of monsters or depressing images. As Blondel remarked, the salutary advice, "mind what you are doing," men never followed more closely than on this occasion.

What does contemporary official medicine have to say on maternal impressions? Not very much, since not much is known with certainty. Fetal psychology is, as the trite pun says, an embryonic field. But it can safely be asserted that the activities of the mother are by no means a matter of indifference to the fetus. This one bathes in hormones secreted by the mother, and those put out during periods of stress undoubtedly affect its physiology. Mothers have always known that a sudden noise, a startling occurrence, can provoke sudden, forceful movements in the being they are carrying in the womb. These reactions are accompanied by changes in fetal heart rhythm and blood pressure. The mother's chronobiological rhythms, her physiological variations, clearly affect the unborn, and the prenatal perception of stimuli have consequences worthy of being studied in detail. It is seriously hypothesized that predisposition to some diseases, including diabetes, stroke, and arteriosclerosis, may start before birth by a process known as "fetal programming."[18] We are closer to agreeing with uncle Toby in Laurence Sterne's immortal

novel, *Tristram Shandy*, when he says: "My Tristram's mis-
fortunes began nine months before ever he came into the
world."

Inside the womb, the fetus sleeps most of the time. It takes
long naps interrupted by short periods of wakefulness, as do
newborn babies. Indeed, the life of the term fetus is not radically different from that of the newly born. We used to think
that being born was the beginning of our lives, the very
moment from which the clock started ticking for us, the mile-
stone that marked the initiation of our existence. But it now
appears that it is only a passing event in the continuum of our
lives, and, to believe some specialists, a rather trivial one at
that. As a neurologist put it, from the standpoint of neurolog-
ical development, birth is "uninteresting": not much happens
that was not already happening before emerging to the light.

Apparently a fetus can dream, since it manifests the rapid
eye movements (REM) characteristic of the dreaming state.
What of? We do not know, and cannot at present pretend to
know. Perhaps of the various sensations received. The fetus
hears, and can respond to sound frequencies between 83 Hz
and 5000 Hz (the healthy adult range is beteen 20 Hz and
20,000 Hz, but there is a drop of the upper limit in old age).[19]
By inserting sound-recording devices into the womb, it has
been shown that the noise level there is comparable to the
background noise in an apartment, since the sounds coming
from outside are attenuated by no more than 30 decibels. The
fetus can hear conversations taking place outside. Inside, the
fetal ear picks up the "maternal symphony," avant-garde
music composed of the whooshing of blood circulating in the
maternal blood vessels, the gurgling and rumbling of her

intestines, and the wave-splash of the amniotic fluid. And all
the while in the background, marking a tempo that is now
grave and solemn like reverberations from a tympanum, now
iterative and martial like the tam-tam of a timbrel or a war-
drum, the thumping of the maternal heart races wildly or
slows down, according to her moods.

Most likely the fetus can also taste,[20] since the taste buds
are fully developed by thirteen to fifteen weeks of intrauterine life. The fetus, although toothless, is reputed to have "a
sweet tooth." It swallows more amniotic fluid if this is sweetened by the addition of saccharine, and less if rendered sour.
Just so the newborn sucks more avidly from a sweetened
nipple than from a neutral-tasting one. Most likely, the fetus
can smell. The mother's diet influences the odor of the amniotic fluid, which obstetricians know can smell of garlic, curry,
onion, or other strongly odoriferous edibles. There is some
evidence that the newborn recognizes these foods in the
maternal milk, whose foretaste it enjoyed while still inside
the maternal enclosure. However, it is undetermined whether
the recognition comes from taste or smell, since the amniotic
fluid is swallowed as well as inhaled by the fetus.

Sight is poorly developed before fourteen weeks of intrauterine life. Light stimulation in the very premature newborn baby
may actually do harm. The optic neural apparatus, from the
retina to the brain, is ill equipped to handle visual stimuli at so
early a life-stage. Nevertheless, at twenty-six weeks the fetus
responds to light flashed across the mother's abdomen.[21] Tactile
sensation, in contrast, is truly precocious. It has been known for
some time that the fetus can respond to touch around the mouth
as early as five and one-half weeks of gestation.[22]

A newborn baby seems to prefer the mother's voice to a stranger's, or even the father's, thereby suggesting that at some level the fetus must have "learned" to identify voices. The same conclusion is applicable to non-vocal sounds. A fetus may react to an auditory stimulus the first time, or the first few times it is applied, but with repetition the fetal response abates or disappears, indicating that the fetus has "learned" to identify it. "Learning" is here put in quotation marks, because the word cannot mean the same when applied to fetuses as when used for children or adults. Researchers often prefer to use the term "habituation," which does not prejudge on the amount of conscious awareness that is present.[23] But even if the recognition response is purely automatic, reflex-like, it is needful to acknowledge that some form of memory is being manifested.

It is one thing to admit that the unborn can see, hear, taste, memorize, and exhibit some form of rudimentary learning; it is quite another to assent to the unfounded proposition that maternal impressions can actually shape the personality or the physique of the unborn. A tranquil, healthy, well cared for gestation has the best chances of issuing in a healthy and happy child. But efforts to improve the intelligence, the beauty, or the character of the descendants simply by securing maternal well being, have not uncommonly been thwarted. As Shakespeare put it, "Good wombs have borne bad sons." (*Tempest* I, ii, 120).

Regardless of our scientific advances, false belief, myth, and groundless, orally transmitted lore continue to survive. As late as the end of the nineteenth century and early part of the twentieth, well-credentialed members of the medical profession were convinced that maternal impressions could affect the physical and mental characteristics of the fetus. The *Journal of the American Medical Association*, in its issue of November 14, 1896, published a report of a complex instance of this pathology. A pregnant woman was frightened by a dog, and gave birth to a girl possessed of an uncontrollable fear of dogs. "Anything in the canine race, even the picture of a dog would distress her."

But the story does not end here. The girl grew to womanhood, became pregnant, and, like her mother, was severely frightened while in that condition by a ferocious dog that bit her. The shock was too great: she miscarried, and the doctor who took care of her—and had formerly cared for her mother—came to examine the aborted fetus. Thoroughly infused by the scientific spirit, the doctor examined the abortus, and took it away with him (those were happier days, when physicians were exempt from the fear of being sued). He made sure that no one would see it, for, O surprise!, its skull was remarkably dog-like. The fact was duly noted in a conference that the physician delivered at the Chicago Medical Society, where he admonished his learned audience with these words: ". . . those who believe in the transmission of maternal impressions, will get some consolation from examining these specimens, and those who believe such results happen as mere coincidences, will have to account for this freak as best they can . . ."

To my eye, one of the most colorful examples of maternal impression believed to have shaped the son's character is of historical interest. The unfortunate son was James I, king of England. This monarch is said to have grown to be a niddering man, who could not see a dagger or a sword without breaking into a cold sweat, and sometimes fainting. But the general belief was, his timorousness and craven spirit were only the consequence of his mother having been frightened when she was carrying him in her womb.

His mother was Mary Stuart (1542-1587). She was the grand-niece of Henry VIII, and the only child of James V of Scotland and his French wife, Mary of Guise. Many a biographer has raised Mary Stuart, a tall, slender, attractive woman, to the status of a romantic and tragic queen. The main facts of her life are well known. After she became a widow upon the death of Francis I of France, she left this country, where she was raised, to return to Scotland. Here, her personal blend of blithesomeness, Gallic urbaneness and *joie de vivre*, sat poorly. Her ill-advised marriage to her no-good cousin, the earl of Darnley, did not make things better. She was drawn into a maelstrom of bitter resentment and adversarial politics that eventually tossed her to the executioner's block.

She was dining one evening in the company of her secretary and confidant, the Italian David Rizzio (also spelled Riccio), when assassins, poniard in hand, broke into her chamber. They made for the man, who was no warrior and had no way to escape. Screaming dolefully "Mercy! Mercy!", the victim desperately clung to the queen's knees. But there was no abating the furor of the killers, Scottish nobles led by Darnley who alleged—with what justification, historians will forever debate—an affront to his conjugal honor. It is impossible to describe the terror that must have seized the pregnant queen on that baneful occasion. Merely to recall it is painful: the candles extinguished, the tables overturned, the dishes broken, the curtains rent by a desperate man being immolated; and all this mingled with the howling, the horrid screaming of both Rizzio and the Queen.

She gave birth to James I who, contrary to what many expected, showed no scratches or skin lacerations on coming to the world. But he soon became a "scaredy cat." He could not stand the sight of an unsheathed dagger or sword. The terrifying experience of his mother was universally blamed for the pusillanimous temper of her royal son. The psychology of later ages might have passed a different opinion.

There was no dearth of possible causes. James was raised by domestics that were mortal enemies of his mother, and who relished repeating in front of him the details of the nefarious and bloody end of Rizzio, and later the no less barbarous end of the young king's father. For Darnley died strangled, and, doleful to retell, Mary married the chief suspect, Bothwell. As if this were not enough, the prince had a pedant tutor and a nurse who treated him unlovingly, and who ensured his obedience chiefly by fear. These personages were instrumental in the design of a coin that was minted in honor of the king. His name was inscribed on one face, but on the reverse appeared a sword suspended in the center, with the words: *"Pro me, si mereo; si non, in me"* ("For me, if I deserve it; if not, into me"). Through the ill will of his tutor, and later of count Bothwell, he was exposed to many dangers and suffered flagrant disaffection; and to top it all he had the misfortune of learning of the cruel end that his mother had to go through.

Verily, the role of maternal impressions does not seem to us, in the present age, of much import in shaping the character of kings (or plebeians, for that matter). It certainly seemed central to the men who lived before us. But, as Richard Lewontin[24] has elegantly said, what we have gone through since Darwin, is not just a revolution of our knowledge of biology, but "a radical epistemologic break with the past." Evolutionary theory changed fundamentally the way we look at the transmission of characteristics from parents to offspring.

There is a certain melancholy in the modern concept of analytical biology. Many of the features that we transmit to the offspring reside in the genes, and we cannot modify them, no matter what we do. Consider our frustration: we respond with unwavering effort to external challenges, and we hope that our conquests and acquirements will help our descendants. All to no avail. The features that we acquire through painful striving we cannot bequeath. Changes in our genes, *mutations*, take place in an entirely fortuitous, haphazard fashion. Some are good, and some bad. Those of our descendants who get the good ones, *i.e.*, the genes that enhance fitness for survival, may be said to have hit the lucky number in this lottery: they will survive. Those who do not, will be mowed down by the Grim Reaper, unfeeling and incorruptible hireling at the service of natural selection.

Before Being Born, You
Must Take Sides

THE RIGORS OF MEDICAL TRAINING HAVE BEEN TOLD many times. Whether the style of epic, dirge, or satire best fits these narratives, I do not wish to consider now. Here, I merely evoke a scene almost forty years in the past, when I was an intern in a hospital, and a newly arrived immigrant in the United States of America.

I see myself as I was then: I am apprehensive in a new environment, stressed by continual forced attention to utterances in an unfamiliar language, conscious of my inexperience and limitations, anxious about the need to impress my superiors favorably, fearful of mistakes, uncertain of my future, exhausted by overwork, dazed and confused by sleeplessness. And I must tend the sick. The telephone rings at wee hours of the morning, and I rush to the floor. Fortunately, this is my rotation in the obstetrical service, where my awkward steps are guided, and my trembling, inept hands ever sustained, by beneficent guardian angels in the guise of specialized nurses.

The true nature of the old-fashioned internship training—whether character-building experience or quasi-sadistic ritual akin to initiation ceremonies of primitive societies—may be doubtful. But the benevolence of some nurses in this system is beyond doubt. It seemed connatural to them to alleviate suffering wherever it was found: physical or mental, in sick patients or in those of us who, though technically healthy, sorely needed their support and sympathy. As I look back, I am persuaded that only the highest encomium can do justice to these kind women. For although male nurses have always existed, in the obstetrical service they were all women.

The chief obstetrical nurse in the night shift is one of the beneficent fairies. I have been summoned because a woman is about to deliver, and I am the physician on call. In her soft-spoken and efficient customary way, the nurse lets me know the salient facts of the clinical history. The "patient" is a healthy young woman. This is her first child. She is Hispanic, poor, and a single mother, but has regularly attended the outpatient clinic for instruction and prenatal medical surveillance. On the side table stands a card with a colored image of the Holy Child of Atocha and a prayer printed underneath. On her bed, pinned to the pillow case, another card displays the image of Our Lady of Guadalupe in her customary garb, her abdomen girded by a black ribbon that, according to tradition, indicates that she, too, is with child—the Holy Child, of course. Apt image to propitiate an uneventful parturition; for the protectress of the Americas ought to be more efficacious in this regard than those virgins who, like St. Margaret, never knew what it is to be pregnant (a fact that does not prevent many women throughout the Catholic world from fervently imploring, when come to the difficult pass, for her intercession).

I introduce myself, realize she is more comfortable speaking Spanish, and quickly establish a good rapport with her by conversing in this our common language. Seeing that everything is going well, the nurse gives me some indications in her usual discreet way, that is, without appearing to be aware of my ignorance and inexperience, which, however, must be only too plain, and goes off to the nurses' lounge, for a coffee. Her withdrawing is one more mark of her discretion. The birth is anticipated to be a normal event, and the nurse wants to promote my self-confidence. This is to be the first time that I feel I am "in charge" in the delivery room. I am to summon her when the delivery is about to happen. In her experience as seasoned practitioner, this is not to be for some time.

The progress is more rapid than we expected. The uterine contractions are vigorous, and follow each other in close succession. Soon, the dilatation of the cervix is complete, and the baby is engaged in its final phase of descent. Only then do I realize that not all is well. With each contraction the baby's head advances downward, and immediately thereafter retrogresses, as if hindered by some elastic obstacle that first yielded, then sprung back. Under direct vision I discover that this is precisely what is happening. A fleshy band, very much like a strap, is draped across the top of the baby's head. Each forceful uterine contraction propels the fetal body, and rams the head against this band, which is stretched thin; but as soon as the contraction subsides, the band contracts back to its original shape, exactly as an elastic band when the stretching tension ceases, and in doing so, returns the unborn to the place it occupied before the thrust.

I am terrified: there is no better way to put it. I am inexperienced, and I do not know the nature of this pathology, much less what to do. I do not remember reading anything of the sort. To enhance my discomposure, every contraction is accompanied by doleful moans of the patient, who tosses about, haggard, sweaty, struggling, and pained beyond description. I send for help with the greatest dispatch, and my beneficent fairy, in the form of the chief nurse, materializes in minutes, that to me felt like centuries, in the delivery suite. She recognizes the obstacle at a glance, and with a sense of urgency that preserves a good deal of self-command, and by this fact differs essentially from the desperate anguish that racked me, declares that the obstructive band must be severed straight away. Rather, she says that *I* have to sever the obstacle.

The look of puzzlement in my eyes must be obvious, for she gives me precise instructions on how to do this, all the while making it appear as if I had been the initiator of the measure. The procedure is simple, indeed. The fleshy band is firmly secured between two forceps, and divided in the middle. Free from constraint, the baby slides through the birth canal, and emerges almost immediately to the light of day. It is a healthy boy, to the great relief of the exhausted mother, and, truth to tell, to mine in not much smaller measure.

A student of classical antiquity might know that a Roman emperor was born with a band across his head. The historian Aelius Lampridius (fourth century A.D.) first recounted the bizarre phenomenon.[1] According to this chronicler, on the 19th of September of the year 202 of the Christian era, Antonius Diadumenus or Diadematus was born, who eventually was to rule with the titles of *Caesar* and *Princeps Juventutis*, but would later die assassinated by order of Heliogabalus. Lampridius was aware that some children are born in a "caul," that is, the head covered by a cap or bonnet made of placental membranes; for such caps were highly valued in ancient Rome, and midwives sold them to lawyers who believed that this possession would make them more successful in pleading their causes.

Discussions of the so-called "caul" often start by alluding to the ancient Roman historian and his description. However, the historian made it clear that Diadematus "did not have such a bonnet, but a thin diadem, yet so strong that one could not tear it, for it was shared by veins in the fashion of a bowstring" (...*at iste puer pileum non habuit, sed diadema tenue, sed ita forte, ut rumpit non potuerit, venis intercidentibus specie nervi sagittarii*). It was this peculiarity, the headband or diadem, that earned the future emperor the nickname Diadematus, one who wears a diadem. Roman parents named their children according to their physical characteristics, or coincidental occurrences believed to have portentous or foreboding significance. Thus, Caesar, from *caedere*, to cut, is often said to have been so named because he was born through a cut in his mother's abdomen, or "Cesarean" section. Marcus was favored as a name for a child born in March; Tiberius, for one born on the banks of the Tiber; Lucius, in daytime, when there is light (*lux*); Postumus, after the father's death; and so on.

As to the headband that detained the baby of my internship days, it was not a simple strip of placental membranes. Such a one would never have withstood the enormous pressure exerted by the fetal head pushing against it with each mighty uterine contraction. It was, as I found out from my many times blessed head-nurse, a vaginal septum. In effect,

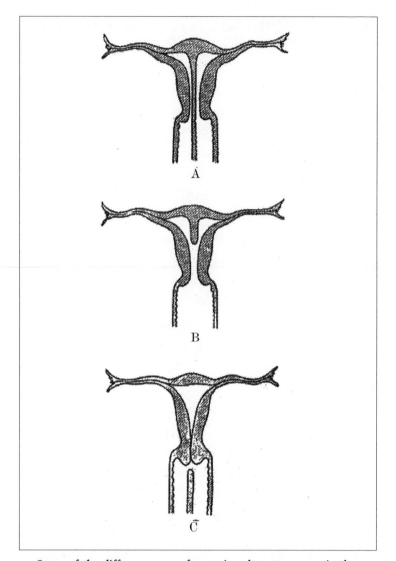

Some of the different types of septation that may occur in the female genital organs. A dividing septum may partition both uterus and vagina (A), part of the uterus only (B), or, as occurred in the case described by the author, the uterus is normal, but the vagina is divided into two cavities by a middle septum (C).

(*From Blair Bell*)

the mother's vagina was divided into two secondary cavities by a tissue septum running front-to-back along the middle; thus partitioned, the vaginal canal could be likened to a double-barreled gun. The fetal head, as soon as it emerged from the womb, encountered the posterior border of this septum, and by exerting a stubborn pressure against it, had flattened it into a strap-like structure. This was the fleshy elastic band that we were obligated to cut off. And, but for the idle nature of most retrospective diagnoses, one might feel inclined to guess that something of the kind must have girded the Roman emperor's head, if Lampridius was correct in asserting that the headband was tough and resilient as a bow-string.

Nor is it a cause for amazement that a woman with a vagina partitioned by a septum should have become pregnant. The internal genital organs arise from paired structures that fuse in the middle during embryonic development. Incomplete fusion is expressed in the persistence of a partitioning wall between the joined embryonic structures. Incomplete fusion may involve only the lower genital tract, or it may extend all the way to the top of the womb. The vaginal septation went unrecognized by the woman of my narrative, her doctor, and her husband. Clearly, it did not interfere with normal sexual activity. The annals of reproductive medicine consign the most bizarre occurrences, and conception and gestation have been known to take place successfully under circumstances more unusual, anomalous, and trying, than those surrounding the patient of my recollection.

After this first experience, I became sensitized to the vagaries of ascertaining the "presenting part," as is said in obstetrics, of the fetus about to become a newborn infant.

There is a proper style, a correct posture to enter into the world, as there is one commanded by etiquette to enter in society or to be admitted to the presence of the exalted. Infractions to the protocol are possible, but are committed at a price: appear uncouth, curtsey at the wrong time, slurp your soup noisily at a dinner, emit digestive or post-digestive noises conspicuously in public, and you may be utterly disgraced. In its progress along the birth canal, the fetus adheres to a demanding postural protocol. This tells the child: first, the longitudinal axis of your body must be vertical, in coincidence with your mother's axis; now extend your head; now flex your neck and trunk; above all, do not stretch your arms!; the head must always come first.

Under normal conditions, the head is the presenting part, that is, the part of the fetal body that is lowest and most anterior in the birth canal during the delivery. The head is thus the tip of the piston in the engine of parturition, the tip of the battering ram that forces a passage forward. The marks of the traumatic progress are imprinted on it. Many a time I watched in surprise a tumefaction that lifted the soft tissues on top of the baby's crown: the hematoma that remained as proof that birth is a battle. The newly born have as much title to exhibit this lump with pride, as a soldier his battle scars. Both have been there and made it back victorious, although some maimed or permanently impaired. Little wonder that the popular imagination has seen the need to create emblems of protection for the newborn. The "caul" is one of them. In effect, as the head is propelled forward, it rends the membranes that enclose the fetus and the amniotic fluid. Very rarely, the tear in the membranes is such that a fragment of these remains attached to the baby's crown, in the manner of a skullcap (if larger, it will resemble a hood or a cape). This is the caul or coif, to which an auspicious significance is most often attributed.

Readers of Dickens know that the caul was supposed to protect against drowning. In the first chapter of *David Copperfield*, the chief protagonist makes it known that he was born so capped, and that the membrane that enveloped him was later advertised for sale in the newspapers, at the low price of fifteen guineas. It was refused by a lawyer who offered a little over two pounds "and the rest in sherry, but declined to be guaranteed from drowning on any higher bargain." Ten years later, Copperfield's caul was put up for a raffle, amidst the misgivings of the young lad upon seeing a part of himself so disposed. The prize was won by an old lady who "never drowned, but died triumphantly in bed, at ninety-two."

In English newspapers, it was not unusual to find advertisements for cauls in good state, directed especially, as one of the ads proclaimed, "to the gentlemen of the navy, and others going long voyages to sea." Thus, in the *Times* of March 9, 1820, a caul was advertised with the publicitary boast that "The efficacy of this wonderful production of nature, in preserving the possessor from all accidents by sea and land, has long been experienced, and is universally acknowledged;" and to reinforce the promotion, the seller offered the reassuring testimony of the "eminent physician who officiated at the birth of the child." In the issue of the *Times* of May 8, 1848, the price of a caul was six guineas. However, the amniotic membranes gradually lost their protective virtues. They were still being sold in the first part of the twentieth century, but by then the prices must have come down, since a newspaper advertisement modestly sets down that no "reasonable offer" will be disregarded, without specifying the amount. In World War I, the threat of death from German submarines, deadly and unseen, transitorily renewed the popularity of the amulet.

The caul's alleged efficacy in protecting against drowning, must have derived from the observation that the fetus lives undamaged while completely submerged in amniotic fluid. But the protection of this membranous object extended to other ills as well, and its varied potency was acknowledged many centuries ago. Thus, in the Middle Ages, a friar was castigated by the ecclesiastical authorities, because he was discovered carrying a caul sewn to the underside of his habit, as protection against black magic.

The Church was forced to combat the superstitious belief in the miraculous protecting power of amniotic membranes. Some had the cauls baptized! Saint Bernardino of Siena (1370-1444) preached against this bizarre custom, whose mere mention he said was "horrible to hear" (*quod horrendum est etiam audire*). The holy man's preaching must have been sorely needed, if one reflects that even priests seemed persuaded of the caul's magical properties. L'Estoile, a Parisian chronicler of the sixteenth century, wrote in his diary in the entry for the twenty-first of September of 1596, that two priests squabbled over the possession of a caul inside the church of the Holy Spirit. The solemnity of the place did not cool their tempers, and they came to blows right in front of the altar, much "to the scandal of all the people."

Protection, however, is a relative concept. An obscure

French poet of the eighteenth century, charged with the composition of an epitaph for a man named Rondon, came up with a salacious verse that, freely translated, may be rendered thus: "Here lies Rondon! Hark the story of his life / When born, the man's head was girth./ At sixty years he took a pretty wife / And died as on the day of his birth." *(Ci-gît Rondon! Voici l'histoire de sa vie, / Le bonhomme était né coiffé; / A soixante ans il prit femme jolie / Et mourut comme il était né).*

By the same token, the mother, who carries the baby completely enveloped in membranes, is not protected herself. In some societies it seemed to be the opposite: the pregnant woman was thought to bring misfortune, and was prevented from entering into certain places, such as mines, barques, or other potentially hazardous sites, on the premise that her presence there might trigger an accident.

It was the opposite of protection that a woman endured, whose child was born in a caul, as mentioned in passing by Richard Burton in his *Anatomy of Melancholy*. The husband, a very jealous man, suspected her of infidelity with a monk that frequented the house, on the basis of the similarity of the child's caul and the monk's hood—a suspicion grounded on the then popular hypothesis that the maternal imagination could modify the fetal anatomical structures.

I never attended a birth of a child born in a caul. This occurrence is very rare. But under the gracious superintendence of my protectress nurse, I exerted myself at recognizing the presenting part. This is done, I was taught, by digital sensation. The gloved fingers of the examiner are introduced in the mother's vaginal tract, and made to feel the top of the baby's skull. In ninety-six percent of all labors, the baby will be lying head down, the back of the head (occiput) forward and to the left in two thirds of the cases, and to the right in the remaining one third. "Can you feel the suture between the parietal bones, running along the midline?" I was asked. I said I did, but I am sure I was not the first apprentice obstetrician who assented out of embarrassment, when in reality I felt no such thing. Afraid to hurt the patient, under conditions that not always respected the privacy of the individual and the modesty of women, and trying to abbreviate as much as possible the uncomfortable maneuver, I felt nothing, or did not know what I was feeling.

The fetal bones are not completely ossified, and the soft, membranous intervals, the *fontanelles* (which Aristotle believed were vents to permit evaporation, otherwise the brain would overheat) can be identified by touch. "Do you feel the posterior fontanelle? Note its triangular shape. Can you follow the midline suture to the anterior fontanelle?" But my fingers felt a fissure here and a ridge there, and these markings seemed to me to be numerous and crisscrossing, and while saying that I felt what I was supposed to feel, inwardly I was convinced that the skull's top was made of innumerable ossicles fitted together, like mosaics in a Byzantine cathedral.

This misconception has a classical lineage. Aristotle, in *Parts of Animals* (653a, 27-29), asserted that the sutures of the skull are more numerous in the male than in the female[2] (of course, since the brains of men, he reasoned, being bigger and more active than those of women, are in need of more ventilation). Admirers of the Stagirite try to excuse this gross mistake by saying that the philosopher must have studied the

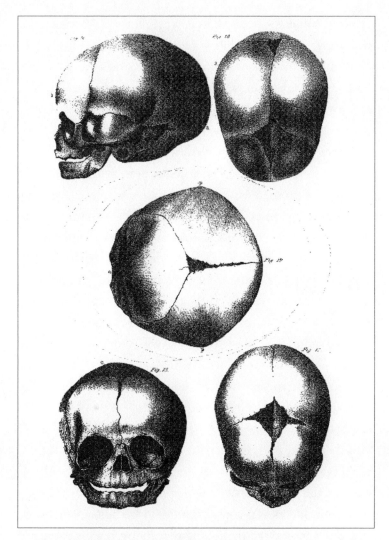

The cranium of a newborn. At birth, the sutures between cranial bones are not yet fused, and large spaces at sites of their confluence remain devoid of bone (*fontanelles*). These "soft spots," covered only by uncalcified membranous tissue, can be identified by palpation. Thus, students of obstetrics learn to determine the position of the unborn child's head by touching its top through vaginal examinations. (*From Ramsbotham, 1847*)

skulls of soldiers killed in battle, where lines of fracture made confusing patterns, and few female specimens. Or else, he may have seen skulls of premature male babies—in which the centers of ossification, which are multiple in the normal state, can give the impression of multiple bones—and skulls of older girls. But the plain fact is that the great philosopher was human, and made a mistake. Aristotle also affirmed that males have more teeth than females. And whereas here, too, partiality for the Stagirite prompts his followers to go searching for excuses, the truth is that there is no justification for so glaring a blunder. For the question of normal dentition is not a subtle theme of metaphysics admitting of various differing conclusions. It is a question of fact, that could have been settled, as Bertrand Russell once put it, "by the simple device of asking Mrs. Aristotle to keep her mouth open while he counted."

In a normal delivery, the fetus will come out head first ("vertex" presentation), with the nape forward and somewhat deviated to the left (left occipito-anterior, or L.O.A. in obstetrical jargon), as if looking toward the right of the mother's back; and a minority of newborns will make their entry into the world in right occipito-anterior position, or R.O.A. Since both positions are considered normal, it seems idle to wonder about any possible hidden meanings of this arrangement. But sidedness is consubstantial to the human condition, and we cannot avoid the feeling that to arrive into the world on one side or the other must have some meaning, albeit one that is perhaps impossible for us to know.

Immanuel Kant[3] devoted an essay, in 1768, to spatial situation and its human significance. He pointed out that we understand directions in space only by reference to our body, and use direction as a characteristic to make distinctions in natural objects or phenomena. The philosopher illustrated this statement with examples that show the pervasive nature of sidedness in our observations of the world. Thus, the hair in the crown of the head grows in a spiral that winds from left to right; hops trace a spiral in the same direction around their poles; beans wind in the opposite direction; and snails secrete shells that, with very few exceptions, coil from left to right (viewed from above, that is, from the apex). This, Kant points out, is a property manifested by snail species regardless of their geographic habitat, whether on the northern or the southern hemisphere of our planet.

To be born inclining to one side or the other would be a matter of complete indifference if the world were neutral in regard to sidedness. But the world, as Kant observes, is not neutral, it "takes sides." It is a partisan world, a polarized world, suffused through and through of a Manicheism that opposes antagonic values and contrary ideas. It is a world that we understand only in terms of perpetual contrast and antonymy: high and low, superior and inferior, front and back, right and left, material and spiritual, past and future, progression and regression. The idea of direction lies ensconced somewhere in this tight tissue of contrasts, and is always overlain with strong emotional tones. For instance, "front" carries a positive connotation, and "back" a negative one. We speak in praise of men with "advanced" ideas and in reproof of those who harbor "backward" notions. "Advance" (from Latin *abante*, from *ab* + *ante*, before), like "advantage," connote ideas of what lies before, what is ahead, in a forward position or direction. Forward is the direction of the gaze, the light-directed sense of sight, which is the fittest instrument of "enlightenment." In contrast, what lies behind is not seen, it is "obscure;" the dorsal world is a blind world; it lies opposite to the gaze, and is, in consequence, recondite, indefinite, spectral, forgotten, and unseemly.

This tense dialectic reaches a high level of expression in the opposition of right and left sidedness. Roger Caillois eloquently called attention to the mystery in this antagonism.[4] For it is easy to see why human beings would tend to acknowledge the preeminence of "upper" over "lower." After all, the constitution of the body leads us to attribute excellence to the upper plane: reasoning, thought, imagination, are the "superior" functions that reside high up in the head; excretion and the elimination of filth are the lot of organs of "lower" anatomical emplacement. Plato, in *Timaeus*, imagined the diaphragm to be a contrivance designed by the gods to separate the noble functions of the upper plane from the life of instincts and ignoble appetites housed in the lower reaches of the body. Hence, it is no surprise that most societies metaphorically refer to all that is ethereal and spiritual as "elevated," and brand all things gross, vile, or vulgar, as "lowly." But why should there be different attributions to the right and the left sides? Nothing in the body would seem to predispose us to favor one side over the other. The human body is, in fact, symmetrical in the sagittal plane. The viscera are exceptions, but the exterior conformation of the body, like its supporting framework, the skeleton—first and last avatars of human corporeality—are symmetrical: one half is equivalent counterpart to the other. And yet, right exerts predominance over left.

Caillois emphasized that this predominance is not simply cultural, for no known human society ever raised the left side to a position of greater importance than the right. Everywhere, it seems, and of all times, the right has been considered majestic, strong, trustworthy. The right hand is the hand of pledges and solemn oaths; the left hand is the hand of deviousness, of under-the-table dealings. Latin *rectus* or *directus*, German *recht*, French *droit*, Spanish *derecho*, Italian *destro*, Greek δεξιός; these words refer not only to side, but to correct or just; they denote what is "right" or "righteous." In some cases, as in *droit* or *derecho*, the word also means the science of jurisprudence. Because no human society ever conferred such high dignity to the left side, Caillois concludes that right-side preference is not cultural, but universal and basic, stemming from some profound, unrevealed cause. But what could be the cause, assuming he was right in his lucubrations?

On a practical level, it makes sense to be born taking sides. For human beings, when they quit the soothing comfort of the maternal enclosure, are not delivered into the arms of a balanced and equanimous Nature. They are dropped into a biased universe with distinct preferences and partialities. In the early embryo, the heart looks like a straight tube, but it soon bends to the left. The intestine, also a straight, narrow cylinder at first, twists to the right (counter-clockwise when viewed frontally). And the brain, though symmetrical, promptly develops functional lateralization, such as right-handedness and speech on the left hemisphere, and "earedness," or "eyedness," on one or the other cerebral hemisphere. All of this apparently controlled by genes conserved through millions of years of evolution.[5] Preferential sidedness is imprinted in the genes, which is to say at the molecular level, in the DNA. Not only in organic molecules, but in crystals and inanimate materials, whose molecular structure is also askew, slanted in "absolute space," as Kant might say, or, in less abstract, easier language, deviated to the right or to the left (*dextro* and *levo* chemical compounds that change the direction of polarized light waves in one direction or the other).

Pliny[6] in his *Natural History* (bk. VII, ch. viii—46), asserted it is the "invariable way of Nature, that human beings should be born head first, and carried to their burial feet first" (*ritus naturae capitae hominem gigni, mos est pedibus efferri*). He seems to have enunciated, perhaps for the first time, the rule of etiquette that governs a proper entrance and a decent exit. For with respect to coming in and coming out of life, the facts compel us to believe there is a proper orientation to the body's axis. At birth, the direction (with respect to the threshold to be crossed) is head-to-feet; at death, it is the opposite, feet first.

In parts of Germany, the person who recovers health or manages to stay alive is reputed "to have given death a pair of shoes" (*dem Tod ein Paar Schuhe schenken*). If a man recovers, he is no longer obligated to go lie in his tomb, shod in "dead man's shoes" *(Totenschuh*, also a word for funeral services).[7]

In America, where those who die a sudden or violent death do so "with their boots on," an ironic euphemism for life's termination is "to go out feet first." One of Grimm's fairy tales, entitled "The Godfather" (*Der Herr Gevatter*) most vividly expresses this idea. A man receives from a mysterious individual, obviously a sorcerer, a flask containing a miraculous potion that cures the sick. Together with the portentous elixir, the recipient gets this admonition: "All you must do is to look and see where death is. If at the head of the bed, the patient will cure. If at the foot, the patient will die." Striking image of the idea that life flows in one direction, cephalad, and death in the opposite direction, feet in front.

There exist, therefore, an axis of life, head-to-feet, and an axis of death, feet-to-head. Those who cross the threshold of life in the wrong position do so at their own peril. In the world of everyday reality, it is true that inversion of the normal vertical axis at the time of birth is a cause of suffering, and sometimes death. Upon inversion, with the legs flexed in the fetal position, it is the hind part of the body, the breech or buttocks, that is lowered foremost in the birth canal. The so-called breech presentation occurs in about 3.5 percent of all deliveries.[8] The figure is higher, about 14 percent, in earlier stages of pregnancy, but the fetus spontaneously reverts to the normal head-first position in many cases. It is as if the unborn knew the dangers it incurred by disobeying the unwritten protocol, and hastened to correct its waywardness. The risks are not negligible. Long-term disability has been reported in 20 percent of all babies delivered by the breech, regardless of the manner of delivery, whether via the natural route or by Cesarean section.[9]

Prevention of complications is the goal of prenatal care. If the malposition of the fetus is diagnosed shortly before labor, the obstetrician tries to correct it. Unfortunately, between ten and thirty percent of breech presentations go undiagnosed until the time of labor . An obstetrical maneuver rectifies the wrong fetal position: the physician places his or her hands over the mother's abdomen, and by exerting pressures in the right places, the fetus is made to roll forward or flip back. This is known as "external version," a skill that may be acquired by all physicians. I confess I never learned it. Excessive timidity kept me from correctly performing any manipulation that required boldness of execution and force of more than gentle magnitude. I pictured the fetus as a precious, exceedingly delicate creature (in this I did not do it justice, for its resilience is considerable), and myself as some sort of malapert interventionist, the proverbial elephant in a china shop.

Oriental medicine may have, here as in other areas, something to contribute. Recent reports indicate that traditional Chinese medicine treats breech presentation by moxibustion, the burning of rolls of the downy covering of leaves of a plant, (moxa is a Japanese term for *Artemisia vulgaris*) on the skin surface, to stimulate certain acupuncture points. Moxa rolls are burned for seven days over an acupuncture point located on the outer corner of the fifth toenail (acupoint BL67 according to the initiates), and a second one-week course is administered if the first one is not effective. A controlled study claimed success in a large number of cases.[10]

Why would stimulation of a point in the skin of a pregnant woman's fifth toe be effective in changing the position of the fetus that she carries in her womb? This is but one among the many puzzles of traditional Oriental medicine. No viable explanation has been found in Western medical thought. However, it is speculated that the mobility of the fetus is somehow enhanced. If so, this would be a method that views the fetus as an individual, and implies its participation in its own deliverance.

Does the fetus also contribute to prolong its own enclaustration in the maternal body? It was believed that to spread its arms was the fetus' way of manifesting its inconformity with its eviction. Indeed, one more protocolary rule that it must follow is to maintain the arms flexed and in contact with its body. When the feet come out first, the arms are extended, instead of remaining juxtaposed to the trunk. This spreading up of the upper limbs is merely the mechanical consequence of the obstacles that the fetus encounters as it exits. But the ancients believed that this was a conscious movement of resistance, by which the unborn tried to hold on tightly to the maternal pelvis, because of fear of coming out. Pliny (*Nat. Hist:* bk. VII, ch. vii-45) says that Marcus Agrippa was born in this fashion, and that the name *Agrippa* conveys the difficulty in being born, for it derives from *aegre partos*, difficult birth.

An ancient idea contended that labor and delivery start because the fetus, upset at months of confinement, decided to quit the maternal enclosure. There is, of course, no scientific evidence in support of this quaint notion, but I cannot help liking it. It confers a measure of autonomy on those not quite in being; it presumes faculties and abilities of control and free will in the nonaged; it empowers the otherwise puny, feeble and defenseless new members of our species. For the moment a human being comes into the world, a rigid code is prescribed to him, or her, with the caveat that it must be obeyed on pain of death or serious disability. Squeezed, pushed, impelled, rammed down, pulled back, deflected here, thrust there, plucked or ejected at last, those being born are passive toys of uncontrollable forces. All they can do is to bend, duck, flex, rotate, or contract the body; —premonition of our life in the world, where adversity makes us stoop, quiver, oscillate, or knuckle under, and we say we are in control of our own destiny.

Not all of us can be like the divine Buddha, who chose the route of his birth (according to Indian tradition, the right side—note, the right—of his mother), and as soon as he was born took seven steps on each of the four directions, and proclaimed: "In the heavens and on earth, only I am the Venerable One" (an expression that has become proverbial in the Far East, where it is used ironically to tease those who vaunt their own superiority).[11] Or better yet, like Zoroaster, who laughed on the very day of his birth, but whose obstetrical "presentation" no midwife or physician could possibly ascertain, because his brain was reputed to be so active, even at birth, that it throbbed, and repulsed the hand that tried to touch his head.

From Dividual to In-Dividual

COME TO THINK OF IT, THE HUMAN STYLE OF REPRO-
duction does not seem all that different from that of
living forms which we stubbornly (and arrogantly)
insist in calling "lower." Marine sponges, hydras, corals,
fungi, and sundry animal species reproduce by simple bud-
ding or fission. A part of the body emits a prolongation, this
excrescence grows bigger, then detaches from its source . . .
and presto! Out of this severed protrusion, a new individual
has formed.

Our much more complicated—and costlier—way of doing
things, namely sexual reproduction, implies also a detachment
from a part of the parent's body. The mature sex cells, or
gametes, must be released from their natural repositories. The
male's gametes are forcefully ejected outward in the semen; the
female's "pop out" periodically from the ovaries, and, less
excitable than their male counterparts, gracefully slide down
the lumen of the Fallopian tubes (which is in continuity with
the outer environment, and is thus, in a way, "outside"). It is
from these detached portions of the parents' bodies, after their
fusion, that a new individual is formed.

The many problems that this mechanism raised never ceased to vex the best minds of the past, and continued to be a source of hopeless frustration until relatively recent times. Who could have imagined that a new individual was formed from detachable living parts of two individuals? This, of course, was impossible. For it would be as much as saying that an individual has split off—a part of it, anyway—and that another individual has done the same thing, in order to furnish the two detachable portions necessary. But this went against the most cherished dogma of what an individual is. As the very etymology of the word clearly expresses it, an individual is what cannot be split off, what is of one piece. The Latin *individuus* means "indivisible" (from *in-*, negative + *dividuus*, divisible). Still today, many dictionaries give "indivisible" as the first acceptation of the term; and also "existing as an indivisible entity or considered as such."

But if an individual cannot divide, there remained the immensely puzzling question of how, then, did human beings manage to reproduce. The learned who tried to give an answer came from either of two warring camps: the one maintained that reproductive power was the privilege of the male, the other affirmed it to be exclusively or primarily a female prerogative. The wrangling between these two factions, rich in colorful incident and outlandish folly, is eminently narrable, and has been told many times. I will not repeat it here. Suffice it to note that when it comes to coveted privilege, the male sex has a tradition of hasty appropriation, not noted for scrupulosity. So it was that for a long time dad claimed greater generative powers—and therefore rights—than mom.

Here, as in so many conceptual matters, Aristotle was largely to blame. His authority was immense. For many centuries, what the Stagirite said was taken to be the God-given truth, and what he said about women was far from flattering. In the Aristotelic view, Woman was an incomplete man: a being that remained in a state of less than full differentiation, within a spectrum of maturity whose fully accomplished endpoint was represented by maleness. Hence, womanhood was defined as a mode of being characterized by deficiency, incompleteness or shortage; it represented a frustrated or thwarted developmental attainment.

The myth of the Androgyne, as told in Plato's *Banquet*, did not do much for the image of Woman. Recall that here a primordial unity was proposed: both men and women were originally welded together, but scission was brought about by divine surgical intervention. As a result, man and woman, the two halves of the original human, seek each other, ever wishing to fit one into the other, like cogwheels that engage in the corresponding projections or hollows in an engine, thereby to recompose the lost unity. This myth introduces the idea of nostalgia as the basis of romantic love. Lovers yearn for what was and is no more. Perhaps this is why, at least in the West, a grey aura of wistfulness, of sorrowful longing for the unattainable ideal, is found hovering above, or behind, amorous romanticism. Lovers are always "languishing."

On the other hand, the idea of complementariness, as depicted by this myth, does not seem to do justice to the rich complexity of amorous relationships between men and women. It overlooks the constant exchanges, the dynamic interplay of love. Granted that the two halves yearn to come together to recompose the primordial harmony (after all, "harmony" comes from the Greek ἁρμονία, a joining or a joint, or arrangement, similar to ἁρμός, joint, whence the word "arm"). So what? One might as well say that shoes and feet or hands and gloves love each other, since they complement each other so nicely. Or that certain reactive chemical elements have love for each other—as indeed the alchemists and the early chemists proposed in all seriousness—since they seek each other so avidly, to reconstitute the unity of those molecules of which they naturally form part.

Likely to have influenced the ideas on human reproduction was not so much Woman's complementariness, as the concept of her secondariness. For the latter found support even in Holy Scripture: Adam was first, Eve came second. The patriarchal society needed no more; the subordination of women was a facile inference from the sacred text. Not that there was a dearth of appropriate rejoinders. In the *Colloquium Between the Philosopher and the Newly Delivered Woman*, by Erasmus of Rotterdam,[1] the great humanist makes the woman say: "Yes, but Adam was before Christ; and, besides, artists usually do better in their later works . . ." No matter, Adam was first; with respect to man, woman was second.

In a male-dominated society that settled it: he was first; thus, he was the model; she was second; thus, she was an imitation. God created man in His image and semblance. Next, He created woman in the image of man. Woman was an afterthought, a collateral creation. Was not her co-lateral quality well symbolized in her being drawn out from man's side, from his flank? She was a subsidiary element, and as they say in chemical-industrial circles, a "subproduct" of man.

Amidst the confused chorus of voices proclaiming the greater importance of one or the other sex in reproduction, the first sonorous ring of the bell of science was sounded by Gregor Mendel (1822-1884). Born in the Austro-Hungarian empire, in the town of Brno (German *Brünn*, also the birth place of the famous musician Leo Janacek, now in the Czech Republic), Gregor Mendel was first to put biologic inheritance on a solid, scientific base. In two conferences delivered at the Society for Natural History of Brno on February 8 and March 8 of 1865, the concept of genes was outlined for the first time.

Students of biology the world over learn that Mendel worked with plants, and that he was a monk. Monkish patience and humility seem to have been two of his personal qualities. From the latter he derived a fitting disdain for the vainglory of worldly fame; the former was indispensable to the meticulous observations that he did on plants that he grew in his little orchard. On both counts he did outstandingly well. Recording what happened to the plants he crossed, he concluded that there were certain "elements" (the name "gene" had not been coined yet) in the parent cells, *i.e.*, the gametes, that interacted among themselves; that these elements appeared to be particulate, since they remained distinct, separable, without blending with each other; and that their interplay and combination determined the specific characteristics of his plants (for instance, whether the generated plants were tall or dwarfish, the seeds oval or round, the surface of chick peas smooth or wrinkled, and so on).

As to his modesty, it succeeded so well, that his contemporaries and fellow monks never knew that they had a brilliant scientist in their midst. The extraordinary import of Mendel's observations was not widely recognized until his works were pulled out of the dusty shelves in which they rested, unappreciated by generations of mice and spiders, and placed in the hands of scientists who restudied them forty years after his death. Perhaps his modesty worked too well, for even today little is known about Mendel. Mendelianism is the bedrock and foundation of Darwinism, but its eponymous creator occupies a comparatively measly space in the mind of historians of science. Of Darwin we have detailed biographies, one of them by himself, and lavishly illustrated editions of the *Origin of Species*; of Mendel, little more than his correspondence with Karl Nägeli, a botanist capable of assessing the value of the quiet, patient toils that went on in the monastery's garden.

One obvious consequence of Mendelianism was the realization that the both parents contributed equally to the formation of the offspring. Of course, the idea was not new, but for the first time its truth was demonstrated by solid, incontrovertible evidence. The experiments could be repeated; the results could be predicted; and the predictions were remarkably consistent. The ancient debates about the relative importance of the maternal or paternal contribution became absurd. Moreover, the theory was confirmed by the compelling power of mathematics, as Mendel's tenets were formulated in the language of statistics. One had to bow to the ineluctable: father and mother contribute equally to the progeny, each passing on a set of "units" of inheritance, today called genes, of which neither parent contributes more, nor less, than the other.

This is consistent with the idea that the individual does divide or split off. Something of the parental living substance must come off, if the genetic material is to be shared and distributed to the descendants. Therefore, the individual divides, and in a strict sense it is incorrect to speak of "in-dividual." Rather, we ought to say a "dividual," which according to the dictionary means "divisible or divided [. . .], also distributed or shared," as when John Milton writes of the moon that

> "[. . .] she shines
> Revolved on heaven's great axle, and her reign
> With thousand lesser lights *dividual* holds."
> *(Paradise Lost* VII; 380-382)

The French biologist, Albert Jacquard[2] appropriately observes that, considered as a living entity, the individual is, of course, indivisible. But considered as a reproductive entity, he or she is best thought of as a "dividual." And he adds that this simple fact gives the lie to a number of sayings attributed to the popular wisdom. For instance, the quaint notion of "like father, like son" turns out to be a biological absurdity. It is not true that the son is like his father: the son is only one-half like his father. The other half is like his mother. And perhaps he is more like his mother, if certain biologic data are fully applicable to the human subject.

The mother, it turns out, contributes important information even before the female gamete is fecundated. In other words, before the entry of the sperm cell, there are cytoplasmic, non-chromosomal elements of maternal derivation (recall that most cytoplasm is, at the beginning of development, maternal) that are important in the construction of the embryo. Very early on, there is a distribution of molecules in the egg-cell that will influence the embryo's body plan. This arrangement determines the front and the back, and the top and the bottom of the new being. It is as if the mother had the ability to install, even before conception, a system of coordinates or "molecular map" that the embryonic cells will find useful to know where to build a belly and where a back, where a head, and where extremities. Very soon after fertilization, the embryo's genes will determine the manner in which the embryo's body is to be shaped. But at the earliest phases of development, and even before fecundation, there is already an indication of "polarity" in the female gamete. This is spectacularly marked in some animal species, such as amphibians, and less well studied—but undoubtedly present—in mammals.[3]

Next, the genetic apparatus of the embryo goes to work. Its constituent moieties, half from the mother and half from the father, perform their astounding magic, and the result is a new human being. A new living entity —individual ontologically, and "dividual" reproductively. But, in any case, a being like no other. For long before the gametes fuse with each other, Nature had taken provisions to ensure that, with the sole exception of identical twins, the newly fashioned beings should be wholly original, irreplaceable creations. A brief recapitulation of some biologic facts appears necessary to outline the contrivance.

The precursor cells out of which the gametes (both, ovocytes and spermatozoa) are formed, do not differ from the rest of the cells of the organism with respect to their chromosomal number. They have the regular complement proper to our species, namely 46. But chromosomes come in pairs; thus, there are 23 pairs. In other words, each individual chromosome has its "homologue." We do not say its "double," because the two members of the pair are not identical: one came from the father and the other from the mother, of the person producing the gametes. The two chromosomes have the same genes, (say, those that control eye color, blood group, and so on) but in different form (the technical name for the alternative forms in which a gene may exist, is *alleles*).

The genes in a chromosome pair, therefore, are not exact copies of each other. In one member of the pair the genes carry the genetic information of the father, and in the corresponding site of the homologous chromosome those genes exist in the maternal form (the maternal allele).

Now, during the maturation of the precursor cells, the forerunners of the gametes, a peculiar manner of division takes place, by virtue of which the chromosome number is reduced by one-half. Consequently, the mature gametes, sperm and ova, end up with only 23 *individual* chromosomes, not 23 pairs, like the rest of the cells of the body. One chromosome, one member of each pair, is eliminated. But which one? The one that came from the mother or the one that came from the father? The answer is that the elimination is entirely random: now this, now that, without apparent rhyme or reason.

To illustrate this further, let three chromosomes of paternal derivation be called A, B, C, and the homologous chromosomes of maternal origin A', B', C'. Considering the random elimination that took place, the mature gametes could end up having any of the following combinations: ABC, AB'C, ABC', AB'C', A'BC, A'BC', A'B'C, A'B'C'. That is, taking into account only three pairs of chromosomes, the possible combinations are 2 x 2 x 2 = 8 combinations. But there are twenty-three pairs, so that the possible number of combinations is 2 x 2 x 2 . . . twenty-three times! This gives us a very large number, which the savants like to express as 2^{23} = 8.4 x 10^6. Thus, the number of genetically different gametes is so vast, that it is almost impossible for two gametes to have the same genetic constitution (and, moreover, they come together at random). Two human beings generated by sexual reproduction never have the identical genetic makeup. Each one is an original creation. The sole exception is identical twinning, in which the fertilized egg splits in two during a precocious phase of its development.

By itself, the above described mechanism might have been sufficient to ensure that no two sexually generated individuals should ever be formed with the same genetic constitution. Yet, it is not the only agency by which our uniqueness is secured. There is a time during the maturation of gametes, when the chromosomes that make up a pair are seen to come together, and actually to contact each other. It is during this time that fragments of the DNA of the chromosomes thus coupled are actively exchanged between the members of the pair. This phenomenon, called "genetic recombination," determines that genes of maternal and paternal origin end up located in the same chromosome. It is estimated that two or three recombinations take place per chromosome pair. The result is a veritable commingling and reshuffling of the genes of the progenitors—both, father and mother—of the person who is producing the gametes.

It is easy to see that these facts of biology roundly confound the pretensions of "blue blood." (Indeed, blood used to be the substratum on which the ignorance of past ages based the alleged personal excellence of the chosen few). Common sense always argued against the extension of privileges down the generations, from those who earned them by personal merit to those who enjoyed them simply by being born. But only a supine ignorance of biology can explain the conceit of those whose pride of the feats of their remote ancestors deludes them into thinking that personal excellence comes down to them "in the genes." Modern biology shows that the shuffling and reshuffling of genes is such that, in the span of a few generations, the arrangement and distribution of a man's genes would differ greatly from that of his illustrious ancestor; so much, in fact, that from a genetic standpoint he might as well be unrelated to the admired forebear.

In the West, absurdity was pushed to the limit, for tradition bestowed higher respect upon descendants of the oldest lineage, as if the ancestors' prowess shone brighter in proportion as the dust of ages thickened over it. Surely, common sense sanctions the attitude expressed by a personage of the eighteenth century Spanish writer José Cadalso (1741-1782) who says: "Hereditary nobility is the vanity that I base upon the fact that eight hundred years before my birth, a man died whose name was the same as mine, and who was a good man, even though I may be a good-for-nothing."[4]

Modern biology also underscores the role of the accidental in our coming to be. Shuffling and reshuffling of genes, later compounded by genetic recombination, inevitably brings to mind the shuffling of a deck of playing cards, whose random arrangement is compounded further as the shuffled deck is parted into several piles that are joined at random once more. An element of pure chance, as in gambling, looms large at our conception. Hence the ancient, steadfast rapport between childbirth and astrology. An engraving from the Renaissance shows, in one half of the illustration a parturient woman in bed, attended by the midwife; on the other half, one sees two men by an open window at the end of the room, peering intently at the sky: they are the infant's father and the consultant astrologist, who points out with extended arm to the constellations in the firmament. All men would like to read the cryptic influences that control their individual fate. Occultists pretend that the cipher is locked in the innumerable circumstances that surround the moment of our birth: the position of the stars, the direction of the wind, the sounds in the air, the auspicious or baneful forebodings in a multitude of events of arcane symbolism, which they pretend to understand. Had we been born at a different time or place, perhaps only minutes before or moments after the actual timing of our birth, the million determining influences would have changed, and our fate would have been different. Happy or sorrowful as our lot may be, there is nothing we can do to change it; for in this matter, as in so many others, we are at the mercy of the accidental. Nor can we escape its empire without ceasing to be who we are, as the following example makes clear

Imagine a hypothetical situation in which a young woman is advised against pregnancy. She has a transmissible infection, or is taking drugs potentially harmful to the fetus. The doctors' warning is only temporary: if she waits for the infection to subside, or the effects of the drugs to dissipate,

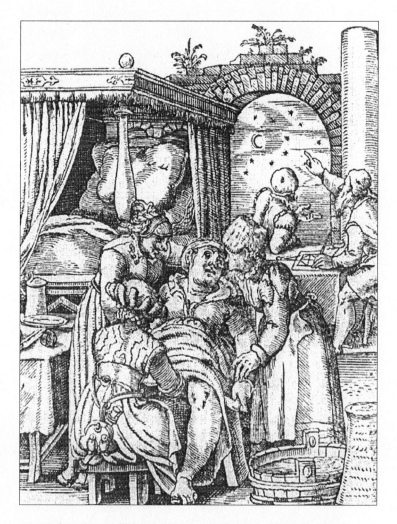

Birth and Astrology. XVI century engraving, showing a woman in labor in the sitting position, attended by a midwife and other women. In the background, a man, presumably the father, consults with an astrologist; both look at the sky, where the arrangement of the stars supposedly will determine the future course of the newborn infant's life.

she will be able to conceive with no danger to the conceptus. But she does not wait, and gives birth to a male infant with serious congenital malformations, whose life is a long recitation of woes, a direct consequence of his physical impairments. He becomes persuaded that his mother's rashness is the cause of his suffering.

At least in the United States, where the courts have heard cases of so-called "wrongful birth," this unfortunate son could bring legal action against his own mother under precisely this rubric. Yet, the possibility of such a suit prospering would be slim. Apart from the fact that, unlike cars, clothes, or household appliances, newly born infants cannot be guaranteed to be free from production defects, what might be the grounds for the hypothetical son's legal suit? If "wrongful birth" is taken to mean that it would have been better not to be conceived, the courts would not hear such allegation. Whether the sum-total of pain and suffering in an individual's life outweighs any positive effects that may attach to being brought into existence, is a metaphysical question, and metaphysics is a forbidden territory for jurists. Important as this question may seem to those concerned, lawyers and judges will appropriately abstain from dealing with problems to which a reasonably straightforward answer cannot be provided. But if the son's allegation is that, had his mother only waited a few weeks or months, he would have been born healthy and spared the harrowing misery that he endured, then the plaintiff's allegation would have no valid grounds. For biology teaches us that, had the mother waited a few months, a different female gamete would have been fecundated by a different spermatozoon. Consequently, a different set of genes would have combined in the conceptus. Therefore, the son would not have been himself, but someone else. And who ever brought a legal suit on the grounds that it is preferable to be someone else?

There are two most prominent genetic effects of sexual reproduction; and, paradoxically, the two run counter to each other. One is in the direction of greater individuality: it makes us unique and irreplaceable. The other goes in the opposite sense: genetics underscores what we have in common with other species. Both are part and parcel of our genetic persona. As to the former, who has not heard that the specific pattern of our genes is today the firmest, most reliable marker of our individuality? Laboratory techniques of molecular biology furnish the most objective, trustworthy sign of personal identity. DNA analysis surpasses fingerprinting for accurate identification of a person. It decides on ascertainment of paternity, when this is in dispute.

The power of the genome! This seal of our individuality can survive long after we have perished, since researchers are able to use the DNA in human remains for their investigations, including that collected from fossilized remnants preserved for thousands of years. Genes spell out the code of our physical attributes, of our unique organic constitution, whose molecular blueprint stays on long after we are gone. Little wonder that in the popular mind DNA occupies the place formerly granted to the soul. No longer do we look to astrology for decipherment of our fate: today, we turn toward the genome. DNA is currently referred to as the key to our identity, the locus of personhood, the map of our existence, the Holy Grail, and the Book of Man.[5]

From this standpoint, sexual "reproduction" is an inadequate word. It evokes the idea of copying, or repetition. But generation is more than mere copying. It is a creative act: the shaping of a new, unprecedented, previously unexampled and thoroughly unique being. "Procreation" better conveys the intended meaning. François Jacob has written that sexual reproduction is an "otherness-making machine" (*machine à faire autre*).[6] For the newly generated being is quite "other": certainly, other than the parents, (as they soon discover, often to their dismay); other than relatives; other than compatriots, coreligionists, or associates; other than anyone else (the only exception, an identical twin). The sexually generated individual was designed by Nature, the "otherness-producing machine," to differ from anyone who is, has been, or will be in the world.

Yet—and this is the paradox of our genetic constitution—together with the mechanisms that underscore the individual's singularity, Nature also proclaims the commonality of all living beings. François Jacob might have done well to propose a *machine à faire du même*, a "sameness-manufacturing machine," or allow that his hypothetical machine could also work in reverse gear, and produce likeness. Here is genuine cause for surprise: that there should be a fundamental unity across the bewildering variety of living beings. No words can express our amazement. What!, the fruit fly and the blue whale, the leopard and the amoeba, all the same? Where is the sameness in the starkly contrasting, utterly diverging species? Still, it is an incontestable, firmly established biologic fact, that a common link—a deep, inalterable nexus of genealogy—joins us all tightly.

Curious to note, the only scientist who, before Darwin, made any attempt to encompass all animal species under a single, overarching conceptual scheme, was Geoffroy Saint-Hillaire (1722-1844), and even he did not elaborate a solid, coherent system. He raised only isolated questions, and proposed some interesting but loose, hypothetical ideas. Nature, he suggested, formed all animals organisms according to a plan that is, at its core, always the same. This plan admitted variation in its details, but its basic foundation remained constant. "Philosophically speaking," he maintained, "there is only one animal," which undergoes innumerable variations. This concept was remarkably penetrating. At a time when all that could be studied of the development of organisms was morphology, his intuition of the unity of all living forms was quite an admirable achievement.

Nineteenth century biologists were surprised to find out that all living organisms are composed of cells. Greater wonder was that the subcellular organization is much the same across the animal kingdom: all cells have organelles; the respective specialized function is the same; the chemical building blocks of the living substance are the same; and metabolic cycles, whole cascades of chemical reactions, are often the same. Essential components are shared from bacteria to elephant, or as biologists say, certain molecules are "highly conserved in evolution." This being so, some similarity of genes was to be expected. But the astonishment of contemporary biologists exceeded all possible description when they saw that genes—the avatars of existence, the supreme tokens of individual identity—were not only similar, but actually interchangeable. The powerful techniques of modern molecular biology permit to cut out a gene—a segment of the DNA molecule—of one animal, and replace it with the homologous sequence of the DNA of another animal of different species—say, mouse to fruit fly. Speechless astonishment, amazement bordering on stupefaction, are expressions that fall short of adequately describing the overwhelming wonder of researchers when they confirmed that the genes so translocated worked well.

The marvels of genetic engineering that stem from this knowledge have been amply publicized. One can, for instance, isolate from spiders the gene that codes for the silk protein, and insert it into the mammary gland cells of goats. The goat's milk thus secreted contains the spider silk protein. This strategy is being pursued by those who attempt to produce spider silk industrially.[7] Human genes inserted into cow's tissue have led to cow's milk that is rich in compounds of medical interest, such as insulin;[8] in sheep, over fifty percent of the proteins can be the product of inserted human genes.[9]

Thus, marked similarities exist in the genes of individuals of different species, and they have been shown actually to work in similar manner. Nevertheless, the total functional effect differs markedly: after all, a spider is a spider and a goat is a goat. To coin a metaphor, the number of instruments is rather limited (a surprise to scientists who elucidated the whole human genome was the relatively low number of genes, much lower than expected), but the musical repertoire is almost limitless. Or we could say that the instruments are much the same, but the music changes infinitely. For this to happen, orchestration is of the essence: winds here, strings there, and the effect on the listener will vary immensely. So with genes in embryonic development: one is active and another repressed; one modulates the next one; or the product of a gene loops back to influence the source whence it originated. And from this knotty, gnarled, devilishly twisted web of actions and interactions, a new individual is gradually shaped.

Nevertheless, the degree to which we share genomic similarities with other members of the animal kingdom, ought to make us pause and reconsider our relationship with other animal species. I say it "ought to," and may I be excused for expressing my skepticism over the possibility that it will do so any time soon. Since genes are the acknowledged repository of biological individuality, the least that can be said is that animals are individuals. We are all related, and this should be sufficient to makes us reconsider our usual relations to animals.

At least one contemporary philosopher, Peter Singer, goes so far as to state that certain animals are, in his carefully laid out definition, "persons," and are entitled to all the respect that personhood demands of us.[10] This certainly sounds odd, but Singer summons impressive arguments to support the existence of "non-human persons." Be that as it may, the sad truth is that our attitude toward our cousins, the animals, has been one of unmitigated war. Worse than the wars engaged against members of our own species, for wars among men are neither universal, nor perpetual, nor accompanied by a licence of unrestricted cruelty.

Let's face it: the work of ethologists, cognitive psychologists, and experts in a variety of disciplines, has shown repeatedly that there is no great, unbridgeable gulf between (human) language and (animal) communication; no impassable gulf between intelligence and instinct; no insurmountable barrier between cultural and natural states. Now the biological sciences reaffirm, at the deepest, most basic level they can attain, namely molecular genetics, our close kinship with all living beings endowed with sensitivity and the capacity to react. But none of these demonstrations, no matter how compelling, will suffice to expunge from the human mind the deep-seated belief in an essential distinction, because, as a distinguished intellectual pointed out, "the difference is metaphysical."[11]

In our multisecular vision, the animal incarnates a brutish, violent or lowly vital pulse, to which human nature opposes the immaterial, divine beauty of reason. Hence our belief that our role is preordained to be domination, as theirs is to be subjection; for intelligence and spirituality must ever prevail over the dark forces of animality. As soon as rational discourse started, language reinforced this rigid antinomy by calling "bestial" or "animal" those impulses that it is best to quell, for the sake of preserving the dignity of the human condition.

May it please God that one day we abandon this stance of superiority, which from remotest antiquity has justified the most sadistic cruelties, and learn to regard animals not as insentient utensils of our will, but as companions in creation. But that day, alas, is not near; nor does the requisite change of heart fall within the purview of biology and biologists.

Crossing the Valley
of the Shadow of Birth

WHOSOEVER WATCHES A HUMAN BIRTH FOR THE FIRST time will long remember the experience. It is a sight not easily forgotten. Trainees in the health sciences have to observe the amazing phenomenon as part of their education. I had never seen one before I attended medical school. Raised in a big city, I had no occasion to see a cow giving birth to her calf, or a mare to her colt; not even a bitch to her puppies. Thus, I was fascinated, and, truth to tell, no little shocked, when the sobering sight of the extraordinary process first unfurled all its forceful, poignant, awesome complexion right before my eyes.

My first experience I can only compare to that of the initiates at the mystery ceremonies of the ancient Greeks. After days of fasting and purification rites, they were led into an imposing temple; and there, amidst the rumor of prayers and chants; awed by the gigantic statue of the tutelary god whose flickering shadow projected over them by the light of torches; with their sensibilities perhaps further stimulated by some psychotropic preparation; the young initiates went into a state of trance. In such a state, according to Aristotle, there could be no learning (*mathein*), but only "experiencing," a sort of hard experience, which the Greeks called *pathein*.[1] Just so: led into the delivery suite for the first time, at the early hours of the morning, overstimulated by coffee, and made to watch the intimidating spectacle of birth, I went into a state that precluded learning. The "pathos" must have been serious, because as a student of obstetrics, my performance was simply "pathetic" (in the sense of pitifully insignificant that the word has acquired of late). I never thought of becoming an obstetrician.

The culture in which I grew up was, I think, inherently adverse to the idea of males embracing the art of midwifery. Never mind that the foremost obstetricians were, and still are, men. That has to do with money, power, prestige, the ascendancy of technology, and a number of factors that are the stays of patriarchy. This, I am afraid, not a burning concern for the health of woman and child, is what historically drew the greatest number of men to the business of delivering babies. There were, of course, some admirable, outstanding, profoundly compassionate physicians. But in man-dominated society women's ills were not the highest preoccupation. I am old enough to remember that, a generation or two ago, men's traditional involvement in the birth process could be called, at best, peripheral. The standard situation was as follows.

As soon as labor started, the husband (even this term is no longer adequate; today it may be best to use "companion") would find some means, in his nervous agitation, to transport the woman to the hospital. There, he would look like the epitome of awkward redundancy. Which is why the nurses would promptly tell him to go home, for no resolution was expected for a certain number of hours. An experienced father anticipated the admonishment, and took his leave before the nurses had a chance to foist their complacency upon him. In any case, the future fathers tenderly assured their spouses that they were in very competent hands, dropped a telephone number at the nurses' desk, and quickly absconded.

In sum, the father's involvement in the momentous occasion consisted in withdrawing to his favorite bar, there to wait for news in an alcoholic daze. The telephone would ring, a voice would say "It's a boy!," and the new father would celebrate by ordering a new round of drinks for the entire room full of cheering customers. If the announcement was of a girl, the mirth was less exuberant or the generous impulse less liberal.

Times have certainly changed. In contrast to those insensitive and misogynous ways, the prospective father is now likely to have attended, in the company of the mother-to-be, months of preparatory classes, such as those of the much vaunted Lamaze course.[2] He probably is persuaded, on the strength of the most authoritative medical opinion, that this way mother and child will fare better, and be less prone to post-partum complications.[3] And if months of concentrating on the anticipated happy event; of scrupulous adherence to muscle-toning and breathing exercises; of listening to counselors who fortify his psychic preparedness; if all this, I say, is not enough to give him the morning sickness, he can always wear the "Empathy Belly.™" This is a device marketed by Birthways Company of Vashon, Washington, that may be strapped to the man's abdomen and its weight progressively increased, so as to reproduce a weight gain of up to thirty-three pounds, or about fifteen kilograms. Thus will the male spouse manifest real empathy toward his pregnant companion. Improved models can simulate fetal kicking and stroking movements, exert bladder pressure that will induce increased frequency of urination, shallow breathing, backaches, changes in sexual ability and self-image, and, as an advertisement from the manufacturer quaintly puts it, "fatigue, irritability, and much more!" Guaranteed, it is said, to enhance warm feeling of solidarity with the female partner in parenting—which, if the company's publicity is to be believed, accounts for the sale of over four thousand "empathy bellies" in the last four years.

However, today's sincere efforts of males to demonstrate understanding and good will toward females do not alter the stark fact that birth has been strictly a woman's affair. And so was the attendance of births in most of the world. Midwives probably always existed, but we know they practiced since biblical times, for they are mentioned in Holy Scripture. In *Genesis* (XXXV, 17-18) it is recorded that Rachel, wife of Jacob, went into labor while journeying to Ephrat, and was attended by a midwife who had soothing words for her while she gave birth to a son.

Another episode related in *Genesis* (XXXVIII, 6-17), this one reading strikingly like a soap opera, underscores the midwife's good sense. In this passage, Tamara impersonates a prostitute, and thus succeeds in enticing her future father-in-law to her bed. The man fails to recognize her in her disguise (or so he said), impregnates her, and out of this union twins are born. The delivery was abnormal, as not uncommonly is the case in multiple births. A hand came out first, but the sagacious midwife solved at one time the obstetrical and the legal problems posed by this complication. The former, by managing to deliver two live twins; the latter, that of establishing the precedence of birth, by tying a ribbon around the presenting hand. In Jewish law at the time, it was a matter of the foremost importance to determine who had been the firstborn, and the midwife found a way to ascertain this accurately and opportunely.

For a long time, physicians believed that to minister to the needs of laboring women was beneath their status. When, centuries later, they saw things differently, it was the members in lowest esteem among their guild who first came into the delivery room, namely the barber-surgeons. Also, a tradition of midwifery barred men from entering the birth chamber; just to see them approaching was considered a bad omen. The only exception was priests, and they were no practical help in the proceedings. But it must be owned that midwives discharged their function admirably well; and their performance is all the more praiseworthy given the difficult circumstances in which they exerted their art.

Imagine the harshness of a medieval woman's lot in a rural area (it is a sad reflection that these conditions are unchanged in many parts of the world). She works from dawn to dusk, often in backbreaking jobs alongside with the men, plowing the land or wielding pick, shovel, or sickle. Perhaps she is assigned to less strenuous but no less exhausting jobs: weeding, reaping, threshing, spreading manure, or tending the garden-plot in which she cultivates potatoes, radishes, lettuce, onions, beets, leeks, beans, and fresh fruits, all of which she sets daily on the table.

Mind you, her work does not end here, although in themselves these chores may be deemed difficult enough to bear. She must still go into the house to cook, and scrub, and sweep, and take care of the children, and look after the animals that share living space with the family. Such a woman must needs be extraordinarily strong and resilient. For such a woman keeps working right up to the very last stages of her pregnancy. It has been known to happen that she is overtaken by strong contractions in the middle of the field, during her fatiguing tasks; and that, the descent of the fetus being rather hasty on account of her strong frame and previous pregnancies—typically she has had many—she has no recourse but to quietly withdraw to some protected, shady spot; and there, unassisted, sweating, moaning, under a blue sky and with the lowing of cattle as background music, she puts the child into the world, letting it fall, so to speak, unto the earth, as the fruit falls from the tree branch when it is ripe and ready.

More often, however, she will deliver at home. Childbirth in this environment is not merely a woman's affair; it is a communal affair. Many female friends come to visit and to participate somehow in the lying-in. They talk to the laboring mother—although in some regions of Europe the custom decreed that they talk among themselves, but not to the parturient woman. The women sit around her bed, chattering animatedly: not in vain this ceremonial visit was called "the cackle" in some areas of Europe, and was regarded an excellent occasion to find out all the current gossip. Virgins are excluded: it is inappropriate for maidens to take part in this custom. Each woman recounts her experiences with child-birth, some talk while sewing or embroidering, others bring in buckets of water, boil water, wash linen, and generally pre-pare what is needed. Some will point out the miraculous power of prayers to St. Margaret, the saint whose interces-sion, although a virgin herself, is sure to guarantee a trouble-free, painless birth. Others will recommend, as more effective than the invocation of the saintly assistance, the wearing of the "eagle-stone," an iron-ore, yellowish stone that is natu-rally cavitated in the center and bears a smaller kernel inside which, when shaken, makes a rattling sound: vivid symbol of the body-within-body nature of the pregnant condition.

Central to this fellowship is the midwife. She is not a "professional" in the modern sense of this word. Rather, she is a friend of the family, a middle-aged or elderly matron per-fectly well integrated in the community. She has no diplomas, and owns but little book learning. What learning she has, she acquired on the job; but assiduous practice, good sense, and the honest desire to help women, often make her the most welcome of beneficial influences. She is expert in distinguish-ing true from false labor pains; knows the best time to bring the woman to the birthing chair, and to rupture the "bag of waters"; realizes the need to discard outrageous superstitious customs, such as the wearing of the husband's pants on the parturient woman's head, or having her walk and jump while wearing his shoes—silly antics that ignorant women often performed on the mistaken belief that they hastened the delivery.

On the other hand, she will not oppose those traditions that are most respected in her native soil, provided only they cause no harm. In areas of rural Russia, the walls display icons, and all the locks of the house must be opened, and even the plaited pigtails of women's hair must be undone. In some parts of the Muslim world, the symbolism of folklore could not be more direct: as soon as the woman goes into labor, the doors of the nearest mosque are open, and the mother-to-be is made to wear an amulet with the first four sentences of the eighty-four Sura of the Koran, the one suggestively known as "The Splitting Asunder." This Sura talks in mystic metaphors of disgorgement and extrusion of the contents of the of the earth's interior, and is therefore uniquely fit to influence the fetal expulsion from its maternal lee.[4]

The midwife is aware of techniques of psychologic suggestion and hypnosis, even though she does not know them by these pompous names. Before the Enlightenment, she was the depositary of whatever practical knowledge of obstetrics and gynecology Greco-Roman antiquity had been able to accumulate. She has something to say about the auspicious or worrisome meaning of the circumstances attending birth; for she has heard that a myriad physical phenomena, by their concomitance with the supreme mystery of childbirth, express an occult relationship that astrologers pretended to understand. And she knows all sorts of effective measures to relieve pain and speed up the delivery. Which is why, no sooner the harsh, tiresome, inevitable hand-to-hand combat between mother and child begins, than she is in command of the strategy. She knows the words that becalm, the concoctions that alleviate pain, the meaning of innumerable birth-related symbols, and the conduct that is best for the woman in confinement.

In the Middle Ages, all this knowledge proved her undo-

ing. For what is one to think of an elderly woman who pre-
pares beverages that bring forth uterine contractions to speed
up delivery, and therefore may be resorted to as abortifa-
cients; who speaks of obscure influences portending future
occurrences for the newly born; whose mere words can abolish pain, and sometimes provoke untold anxiety by announcing deformities in the offspring? What can one think of such
a woman, if not that she is endowed with supernatural powers, and is therefore a sorceress or a witch? From this conclusion, it was an easy transition to suspect that she was the
cause of the very mishaps which she foretold.

When misfortune attended the birth, the need to blame
someone found an easy target in the matron. It was not long
before she was accused of causing congenital malformations
and infant's diseases by what she did, or by what she pur-
posefully avoided doing. Midwives were accused of using the
fat of dead babies to smear the devil's staff, or to add to poi-
sonous brews. Demonologists claimed that midwives made
candles with umbilical cords of dead babies, later to use them
in Satanic rites. The bishop of Chester, in England, saw fit to
command that midwives take oath not to use witchcraft,
invocations, charms, or relics. A city ordinance in Würzburg
in 1555 forbade midwives to keep the placenta, presumably
to curb their evil practices. In Brandenburg, as late as 1711,
a law existed that prohibited them to sell cauls (*i. e.*, pieces of
placental membranes). The criminal laws against witchcraft
were abolished in 1735 and 1736, but by then thirty thousand
witches, many of them midwives, had been put to death.[5]

The lot of midwives improved after the Dark Ages, but
tranquillity was not their mead. They now had to contend

with jealous physicians, who vied with them for patients. Every time financial gain is at stake, we can be sure that there will be pitiless and inflexible scheming. Medical men mounted a campaign of slander against midwifery, tinged with the most malicious exaggerations. And yet, were we to tally the sum-total of mischief inflicted to public health, it is likely that the medical profession, before medicine acquired a solid scientific base, caused far greater maternal-fetal harm than midwifery. For the latter generally was guided by the centuries-old tested experience of many generations of women, unencumbered by grand theoretical schemes; whereas doctors who held diplomas from the universities, steeped in fancy preconceived ideas that adverted more to airy philosophies than to human physiology, were apt to guide their actions by erroneous notions. Midwives were a practical, dedicated, estimable group, and, being mothers themselves, they were genuinely concerned with the well-being of mother and child. Doctors of medicine, when medicine was scarcely different from philosophy, joined ignorance to arrogance, which ever has been a most pernicious combination.

As Nancy Mitford[6] points out in her delightful biography of Louis XIV, during the dawn of the Enlightenment, the late seventeenth and early eighteenth centuries, the chief health hazards were: for women and children, childbirth and babyhood; for men, the battlefield; and for people of all ages, smallpox and other infectious diseases. In contrast, the ailments of old age seem not to have been as prominent. Madame de Ventadour nimbly danced the minuet when she was ninety years old; the duke of Lauzun, whom Louis XIV was going to imprison to prevent him from marrying the

Duchess de Montpensier, indulged in strenuous hunting at eighty-nine; and Madame de Maintenon, first mistress and later secret wife of the Sun-King himself, according to correspondence still extant, complained when she was over seventy years old, that his royal highness insisted in demanding his conjugal rights every day, and sometimes twice a day! But all historians concur in pointing out that infant mortality was appalling. Mitford tells us that merely to see the physician approaching elicited despair, for if the patient had a chance, no matter how slim, of curing spontaneously, the awful purges and copious bleeds that were then standard therapy were sure to gravely worsen the malady. Yet, it was not easy to oppose the physicians' recommendations: an unforgiving society would have deemed the opponents guilty of neglect. If the patient died, a not too uncommon outcome, those who had refused to administer the therapy could be accused of murder.

True, excellent male obstetricians first made their appearance at about that time. In France, François Mauriceau (born in 1637) was responsible for many welcome innovations in obstetrical care. In England, William Smellie, coming to the world sixty years after Mauriceau, did much to furnish obstetrics with a truly scientific foundation. But, if the plaudits of the world were distributed fairly, assuredly not a few matrons dedicated to midwifery throughout history deserved by their actions all the approbation and homage freely bestowed on their male counterparts.

A Roman imperial physician in the fourth century A.D., dedicated his treatise of obstetrics and gynecology to a certain Victoria, whom he called *artis meae dulce ministerium*. ("sweet teacher of my art").[7] But of this, as of many other outstanding women who practiced obstetrics (or medicine, for Roman antiquity did not exclude women from this field), nothing is known.

Louyse Bourgeois, French court midwife, is mentioned in history only because she happened to be in attendance to Marie of Medicis when she gave birth to Louis XIII, and left a vivid, first-hand account of the lying-in, of which all history buffs enjoy the colorful details; but of her skill and knowledge, which must have been considerable in order to have been called to look after the queen, and which she consigned to a treatise on obstetrics of her authorship, scarcely any mention is made in most manuals on the history of medicine.

In the eighteenth century, another French midwife, Marguerite Boursier du Coudray, did for her country such beneficence as might have earned her eternal renown, if only she had shown the good sense of being born a male.[8] After learning the *métier* by the then customary apprenticeship that amounted almost to indentured servitude for six years, she struggled with a male-dominated medical profession, and against most difficult odds succeeded in obtaining royal sponsorship for her educational activities. These consisted in traveling along the length and breadth of France, transmitting to women in the countryside, including the remotest villages, her sound, up-to-date obstetrical knowledge.

Madame du Coudray invented what she called a "machine," actually an anatomical model, a mannikin. It was an upholstered contrivance that represented the feminine pelvis. The skin and soft tissues were made of flesh-colored fabric, stuffed with padding. The bones were, at first, real bones from human skeletons; later, wood and wicker models were used. The various parts were identified by their proper anatomical names. A flexible model of a fetus was constructed, and a later refinement consisted in using sponges drenched in clear or red liquid, which, as the "fetus" descended and compressed them, realistically simulated the spilling of blood or amniotic fluid. The only example of Madame du Coudray's "machine" that still survives is kept at the Flaubert Museum (*Musée Flaubert et d'Histoire de la Médecine, Hôtel-Dieu*) of the city of Rouen.

Today, we tend to think that the invention of an anatomical model is not particularly noteworthy. But, considering that midwives in the remote places that Madame du Coudray visited were for the most part ignorant, uneducated women, many of them illiterate, the instruction that she provided was useful in the extreme. She traveled indefatigably, and wherever she went, her "machine" forcefully depicted, better than any number of lectures could illustrate, or any learned treatise could explicate (and which would have been out of reach for her unschooled audience, anyway), the mechanics of birth. For childbirth is, in very large measure, a problem of mechanics: a large object, the baby must go through difficult obstacles in a precisely defined sequence. For this to occur, both, the passageway and the moving body are subject to considerable physical stress: strong pressures, tensions, frictions, and the corresponding displacements, adjustments and deformations.

Detailed knowledge of the mechanics of this "conflict of space," enables the obstetrician to prudently assist Nature, and to know when overzealous efforts may do more harm than good. Incompetence or neglect during parturition may cause devastating, life-long ills, and provokes grievous sorrow in those afflicted. By replacing obscure superstitions and irrational customs with correct anatomical notions and sound obstetrical practices, Madame du Coudray did incalculable good to the health of her nation. Surely, among the many statues of kings, generals, and other worthies that stand in Parisian parks and plazas, she deserved at least a small commemorative plaque. I know of none; from which I gather that, for society, the sword is mightier than the obstetric forceps or the vaginal speculum.

This and other midwives of the period experienced no universal gratitude. Instead, they tasted frustration on account of the inefficient bureaucracy of the *Ancien Régime*, and unalloyed hatred on the part of the organized medical profession. One can get some idea of the venomous rancor that festered in the breast of medical men (for they were all men), by reading the reference to midwifery in the entry on "parturition" (*accouchement*) in the profoundly influential eighteenth century *Grande Encyclopédie*, under the direction of the famous philosopher and writer Denis Diderot.

Diderot was not the author of this article, which is an egregious example of bitter, slanderous attack. The opening lines ("Prompted by the curiosity to see man's birth . . . after having seen his death time and again . . .") give away the author as a physician, for at that time many physicians were likely never to have seen a birth. Still, that the justly famous opus should have incorporated this piece of outrageous slander, shows the depth of the prejudice against midwives:

> "I [went] to visit one of these women . . . who receive young people seeking instruction in the matter of deliveries, & I saw there examples of inhumanity that would defy

belief in a land of barbarians . . . These midwives, in the hope of attracting the greatest number of spectators, and therefore payers, sent emissaries to announce that they had a woman in labor, whose child with all certainty was coming unnaturally. People arrive; and not to deceive them, they returned the child into the womb and drew it by the feet. I would not dare to say this if I had not been an ocular witness several times, & if the midwife herself had not had the imprudence of confessing it to me, after all the attendees were gone."[9]

Those familiar with the process of childbirth will realize the implausibility of this truculent story. The fact is, the midwives' standard of practice was satisfactory, compared to that of organized medicine. Solid historical research performed by Dorothy Wertz shows that in North America during the early colonial period, when all births were attended by midwives, the results were much less dismal than detractors of midwifery made them appear. Assuming that all deaths of women in the reproductive age (between fifteen and forty-four years) were due to childbirth, still only less than five percent of births would have been lethal to mothers.[10] We would like to think that the progressive wresting of obstetrical practice from midwives and its incorporation into official medicine— controlled by men—was a consequence of scientific advances. Alas, it was not so; determinants much less lofty were at play. In colonial America, of Salem witch trials fame, the Protestant authorities explicitly barred midwives from engaging in "women's lore," meaning magical practices. So divested of their imposing aura, they began losing ascendancy. But the chief cause of their degradation was financial: delivering babies was a lucrative business, and male practitioners wished to corner the market. Records reviewed by Wertz show that the following medical fees were charged during the late eighteenth and early nineteenth centuries : 1 shilling for a tooth extraction; 2 shillings for an average house call; 3 shilling for bleeding ("procedures," as it is now said, were always highly esteemed in the profession on account of their profitability); 12 shillings for setting a fracture; and no less than one pound for delivering a baby, which could turn into a never-to-be-slighted three pounds, if paid by the State.[10] Men were not about to let women take away from them so bountiful a treasure trove.

The displacement of the matrons was accomplished with exemplary finesse. Diverse arguments, of various shades of misogyny, were wielded. It was pointed out that to attend a birth is "messy"; why, with all that blood, secretions and excretions, no refined, educated lady would ever think of engaging in this activity. Every new technical acquisition was deemed inappropriate for women. Thus, the use of obstetrical forceps was unlady-like; moreover, instruments were so designed as to require the sort of physical strength that—it was then thought—women lack.

New techniques and instrumentations were first developed and tried in hospitals, but no well-bred lady of the middle class would be seen in a hospital through most of the nineteenth century; not as staff, and most certainly not as patients. It is well to recall that well into the nineteenth century, only pauper women with complicated pregnancies, or disgraced girls of low social strata with out-of-wedlock pregnancies, or prostitutes, delivered in hospitals. In the United States, it was until after 1890 that hospitals started soliciting paying patients, who received treatment in private wings for the affluent. Before that time, only the most desperate circumstances would have forced a self-respecting woman member of the bourgeoisie into those squalid dens of human abjection.

Aftermath of the Midwives' Deconstruction

Obstetrics eventually came into its own as a science-based medical discipline. It was, in the United States, the first major medical specialty that offered certification through National Board examinations. Specialized resident physician training was soon set up. In the 1930s, committees were first established to investigate maternal deaths in childbirth, which, being largely preventable, are a good index of the quality of health care in a community. But it seems that before all his took place, male physicians had very effectively eliminated the competition.

However, it would be unfair to say that in elbowing out females men were actuated by nothing but invidiousness and ill will. It is perhaps a truism, but it bears repeating, that human beings are products of their own society; and doctors only reflected the unabashedly misogynous collective attitude prevalent in by-gone eras.

It was a paternalistic misogyny, mind you, that cloaked its message in a language of lyrical tenderness. Woman was a frail flower of compassion, beneficence, and love. Her mind was made for soft impressions; the very sound of her voice conveyed this inner delicate harmony. Anyone could see that a graceful mouth, and soft, beauteous limbs, and a constitu-

tion more lovely than fearsome, were made not for hateful
strife, but for love and friendship. But, this flattering depiction once completed, the question was: what is such a lovely
being doing in a hospital, anyway? It is not her role to handle surgical or obstetrical instruments!

In the nineteenth century, an author extolled the hand
that rocks the cradle, and finished his lyrical flight admon-
ishing women: "You who assist us in the cradle and at the
edge of the tomb! Be forever what Nature made you . . .
Never usurp from us the empire that you will always have;
your power resides entirely within your weakness."[11] And
another writer, well into the nineteenth century, plainly
declares: "Man is well pleased with a courageous independ-
ence, whereas woman prefers a sweet servitude."[12]

Men arrived into the business of caring for mother and
child with the hefty baggage of prejudice and received misconception proper to their times. Not the least of the warped
views were the absurd, conflicted views on women and sex.
In the eighteenth century, a book was published in France,
whose title, freely translated, was "On the Indecency of Men
Assisting Women in Labor."[13] Its author was a prominent
physician, who had been dean of the Faculty of Medicine in
Paris. Thus, the book reflected what must have been a very
widespread sentiment.

Direct visualization of the female external genital organs
had long been, for men, more than a simple cultural interdiction: it was a taboo, an atavistic, irrational, emotion-laden
restriction. Hence the myths in which a male voyeur, like
Tiresias, is punished with blindness for his visual transgres-
sion. Generations of men had thrown dark veils, one after

another, to conceal those parts that a colorful medico, Nicolas Venette (1633-1698), called "Nature, because all men originate therefrom," and which "are the cause of most of our chagrins as well as our pleasures; and I dare say that most of the disorders that ever were in the world, and which continue to appear every day, come from those parts."[14] Venette concluded that genital hair growth at puberty is Nature's way to "put a veil upon the privy parts of both sexes, to signify that modesty and honor must establish thither their main abode."

It is paradoxical that the takeover of the practice of obstetrics and gynecology by men was carried out when pruriency and puritanism were at their peak. Even today, despite our much freer mores, a young male medical student who must approach the physical examination of women's reproductive organs for the first time, cannot avoid the obscure sense that he breaks a formal prohibition; the consciousness, however dim or inchoate, that his acts are an open violation of decency; that he is the agent of an intrusion that goes squarely against women's modesty, and commits thus a misdemeanor for which some punishment must exist. In time, the medical man will abstract his scientific interest from any distracting notions or confused feelings. Aided by reiterated experience, he succeeds in drawing his mind away from culturally determined anxiety and focusing on the pathology. But his first experience is troubling. It is akin to that of the eighteenth century American medical graduate who is asked to examine a pregnant woman by introducing his fingers through her vaginal canal, in order to determine the position of the fetus. He approaches her trembling, sweaty, nervous, confused, and after performing the maneuver concludes:

> ". . . whether it was head or breech, hand or foot, man or
> monkey that was defended from my uninstructed finger by
> all the distended membranes, I was as ignorant, with all my
> learning, as the fetus itself that was making all the fuss."[15]

It is not surprising, in view of the aforesaid, that many techniques and procedures that became standard in obstetrics were not the result of deliberate study and careful clinical observations, but grew out of sheer prejudice,—the latter often times in ignorance tinct. Such is clearly the case with the posture of the woman in travail. In many areas of the world, she instinctively adopts the kneeling position; others prefer to be sitting, or squatting; very few lie supine.[16] But, the lack of any obvious benefit to the birth process notwithstanding, in most hospitals of the Western world the woman is made to lie on her back. Enquiry into the reasons for adopting certain positions during labor led the enquirers to conclude that medical or scientific considerations were not a factor.[17] Instead, the prurience and neuroticism of the male practitioners, and a pharisaic conventional morality, led them to advocate such birthing postures as seemed, to their eyes, less "indecent." As one of them put it, considering how far the modesty of true ladies is carried, "and reflecting on their extreme delicacy and the reserved character of their manners and customs, we are rather led to think that the lateral position which prevents them looking at the accoucheur in the face, has been chosen to gratify and save them from unpleasant feelings."[18]

Be that as it may, in most industrialized societies, delivering babies turned into a male-dominated activity after having been for centuries an almost exclusively female occupation.

And it ended looking very different from what it had been in the past; the changes radically altered both its practice and its theory. Much of the traditional midwives' knowledge, the good with the bad, was lost. Obstetrics became increasingly scientific and technologic. Every birth was regarded as a pathologic phenomenon. One of the most influential textbooks of obstetrics, by Dr. J. De Lee, perhaps the foremost authority worldwide in the first half of the twentieth century,[19] unambiguously stated that ". . . derangements so slight as to be of little consequence under ordinary circumstances, may readily give rise to pathological conditions which seriously threaten the life of the mother, the child, or both." It might seem odd, sagaciously commented Dr. De Lee and his followers, that pregnancy and delivery should be called pathologic, but impartial scientific observation of the risks involved reinforced the impression that it was "decidedly a disease, a pathologic process." In other words, accident, disability and death lie in ambush behind every birth, like the adder behind the flower.

Therefore, like all life-threatening diseases, childbirth had to be taken care of in a hospital. Childbirth was in essence like appendicitis, typhoid fever, or pneumonia. The early promotion of this idea had nothing to envy the sophistication later attained in Madison Avenue: "If you developed appendicitis, you would not think of having an appendectomy lying on your kitchen table. So why settle for delivering a baby at home?" Why, indeed? So thorough and so rapid was the success of organized medicine in persuading the public, that in the United States, where only five percent of women delivered in a hospital in 1900, by the 1930s close to eighty percent of all women in urban areas were delivering in hospitals. The reasons were many, but the undeniable progress of medical knowledge must be counted among the main ones. The hospitals' sinister reputation as ante-chambers of death had been due in large measure to the appallingly high number of (puerperal) infections, but by the close of the nineteenth century these were under control. Moreover, the spectacular advances of medical science in general could not be gainsaid: better anesthesia, improved pain control, accurate diagnostic tests, antibiotics, and so on. And then, that Americans have long stood in reverential awe of scientific-technological advances scarcely needs reiteration. The fact is, with the exception of distant rural areas, virtually the entire population looked to the hospital, not the home, as the most appropriate venue for babies to come into the world.

The untoward consequences of this change are now well known. They were outlined in two epoch-making books of keenly perceptive social criticism, although differing markedly in style: Richard Wertz and Dorothy Wertz's *Lying-In*,[20] and Jessica Mitford's *The American Way of Birth*.[21] Many other publications have been critical of specific measures implemented in the care of pregnant women during labor (*i.e.*, sedation, cesarean section, forceps, and so on), or of the motives of the medical profession in this connection.[22] It is important to bear in mind, however, that the transfer from home care with traditional measures, to technology-oriented delivery in a hospital, was implemented as much by the persuasion and influence of the medical profession, as by the unwavering, insistent demands of the public, who thought it unconscionable that physicians should withhold newly developed measures to alleviate the ills annexed to childbirth, especially the relief of pain.[23]

All critics agreed that a major untoward effect was the dehumanization of the birth process. To accommodate millions of women in hospitals, the obstetrics ward had to be transformed into something that resembled, as the trite saying puts it, the assembly line in a factory.

Picture the woman in labor in a modern-day hospital: draped and strapped to a bed, her legs up in the air in the so-called "lithotomy position" (feet fixed on the bed's stirrups, legs spread apart). She is attended by a harried resident physician who examines her, after an intern has taken her clinical history; and a laboratory technician a blood sample; and an orderly wheeled her to the radiology area, where another technician mobilized her as was deemed appropriate; and a radiologist interpreted the images obtained from her abdomen; and a solicitous nurse set up the intravenous solution . . . As she reflects on this division of labor (no pun intended), in which each worker is interested in only one part of her body, or one aspect of her care, will she not feel a little forlorn, and conclude that there is, after all, more than a slight resemblance between the efficient, impersonal way she is being treated, and the slick, profit-oriented techniques of production in an assembly line?

Will she not be entitled to feel that something valuable was lost when the traditional ways were given up? There is no question of a true camaraderie and a sense of fellowship with other women; no feeling of belonging to a large social group. The presence of the husband, when available, is not an adequate substitute; nor is he welcome inside the delivery suite in all cases. And there is no sympathetic midwife, either.

Still, there was supposed to be the consoling, reassuring presence of the physician. For in gaining control of the monopoly of obstetrical care, the physician set himself up as counselor, guide, and sage: he was purported to be the quintessential father figure; his ministrations ensured that a healthy offspring join the family and strengthen it; and he held the key to the reproductive future of that family, advising the woman on what to do in her reproductive life. Only we know very well what happened to the much vaunted doctor-patient relationship of yore. The old, wise practitioner became much too busy to be able to stand alongside his patient during the many hours of her labor. As to his young stand-in, when interrogated about his rapport with the ladies in travail, he is apt to answer in the manner of a fourth-year resident physician in the obstetric ward of a large hospital, who was quoted as saying: "We shave 'em, prep 'em, we hook 'em up to the I.V, and administer sedation. We deliver the baby, it goes to the nursery, and the mother goes to her room. There is no room for niceties around here. We just move 'em right through . . ."[24]

It is not surprising that many women rebelled against this state of affairs. Starting in the nineteen-sixties, and steeled by a reinvigorated feminist ideology, many women rejected hospital care and all it entailed. They rejected the basic definitions constructed by the biomedical establishment, and the value judgments they carried. They rejected most pre-natal training methods, as paternalistic and punitive (if the right results are not obtained, the blame is placed squarely on the woman, who "failed to comply as expected"). They infused new vigor in the practice of midwifery, whose much needed empathy for women they extolled. They protested against the concept that pregnancy is a disease prone to deadly complications, asserting it is healthy and safe. Wherefore they saw no need to go to the hospital, and preferred to give birth at home, attended by family, friends, and midwife, since this is the most nurturing environment for mother and child.

The basic stance of these women has been called "holistic," because it views mother and fetus as one. In contrast, biomedical technology is analytic, that is, it approaches problems by dissecting them, by teasing them out into simpler components, as scientists are wont to do, in order to facilitate understanding. So it is that every form of biomedical technology, from simple ultrasound imaging to complex DNA molecular studies, apart from yielding valuable clinical information, serves to emphasize the separate identity of mother and child.

Adherents of the "holistic" ideology thus stand in opposition to a "technocratic" faction that places its trust in the progress of biomedical science and technology. The former group believes that technology is not to be trusted, since it turns women into things; and by obtunding consciousness makes it impossible for women to find any meaning in childbirth. Birth, they maintain, is essentially unpredictable, a sensuous experience; even, some have contended, an inherently sexual one.[25]

The technocratic partisans retort that technology is liberating; that by freeing women from pain it makes their lives richer, enabling them to experience birth fully as their own creative act.

Votaries of the holistic persuasion speak of childbirth in poetical metaphors, for they claim that only the language of poetry comes close to expressing their meaning: birth is a journey, a voyage that human beings must complete (many, although in the world, were never born: they were abruptly pulled by gloved hands from the maternal enclosure, before completing the journey); and labor is a force of Nature: a mighty wave that envelops the mother, who, if she is wise, ought not to oppose it, but let herself go in the direction of the resistless force.

Not so, reply believers in technocracy. Nature can be, and must be, controlled. Biomedical science can prevent women from falling into the abyss of awesome, unopposable biologic forces, thereby losing the noblest strands of their humanity. Only by preserving an even-keeled awareness shall they become fit to experience with utmost lucidity love, fear, joy, and those transcending, ineffable feelings that some describe. Only the woman in command of her inner self can fully participate in the experience of birth.

These two perspectives on childbirth continue their dueling, in modified form, down to our day. It is fit that it be so; for they represent the obverse and reverse of the human spirit. The technocratic vision embodies our faith in the sovereign powers of the intellect; it inspires us with the conviction that Nature can be understood and regulated. The holistic view embodies our affective side, that part of our being rooted in the subsoil of emotion, whence sprouts all that is warmth, lyricism, and irrepressible sensuous energy. In one of his lyrical flights, and with an off-handedness that classical scholars might find unacceptable, Nietzsche called these two tendencies Apollinian and Dyonisiac, respectively. The former he linked to Apollo, the sun-god of the Greeks, who saw things present and future clearly and distinctly; the god of light. The technocratic viewpoint is Apollinian, because it is eminently rational, and reason allows us to "foresee" things, and enables perceptions that are clear, unambiguous, distinct, and reproducible in all observers.

In contrast, the god Dyonisus symbolized for Nietzsche all that eludes a rational, systematic, orderly manner of thought. The holistic view of childbirth he would have thought, no doubt, Dionysian. The ancient Dionysian cult was ecstatic, orgiastic, hallucinatory, and explosive: the god's ceremonial chariot was represented as covered with flowers and garlands, pulled in ceremonial processions by panthers and tigers that were harnessed to it, like beasts of burden. As it approached, his votaries fell to the ground convulsing, awe-struck , smitten by the terrible divine refulgence: he was the god of madness and ecstasy, but also a mighty leveling force. Before him, the artificial barriers between man and man dissolved in a preternatural form of chaos that was, at the same time, a harmony; by his rapture conventions vanished, and the impositions of necessity became meaningless.

Need we say that both perspectives are necessary? As in any quandary of human life, a mid-course, if possible, is best. A holistic fundamentalism is rash, retrogressive, and undesirable. Only an obscurantist fanatic would deny the benefits of antisepsis, analgesia, early diagnosis of complications, and other boons of scientific progress. Most women agree that their reproductive lives were made happier, and their obstetrical experience less grievous, than those of their grandmothers, thanks to these advances.

On the other hand, a technocratic approach by itself, unregulated and unsupervised, is apt to incur a dehumanizing excess. Left to its own devices, as the experience of industrialized societies well shows, it will end up creating an unfeeling atmosphere that is repugnant to human dignity. Fortunately, the holistic view exists, which will countervail technocratic excess. This, indeed, may be its reason for existing: to check or attenuate, if not to cancel or rescind, by means of a poetic turn of mind, the rash call to march ahead on the route of technological progress without asking why or wherefore.

Coda

It seemed implausible and misleading to end these considerations here. For the disputation between advocates and detractors of birth-related technology, a debate apparently so important in industrialized societies, is moot elsewhere, which is to say in most of the world. Each year, half a million women die during labor, or in the period immediately preceding or following delivery. It is as if there occurred a plane crash every four hours, involving a modern jet fully loaded with two hundred and fifty passengers, all of them pregnant women.[26] That most of these deaths are entirely preventable is clear when one contrasts these appalling figures with the obstetrical mortality rate of countries in the industrialized West: one hundred and twenty in France, and barely sixty in Finland.

What possible resonance could have the conflict of technocratic and holistic perspectives for most mothers in rural Bolivia, Senegal, Bangladesh, or Burkina Faso? In Mali, 8,000 women die in labor for every 350,000 births.[27] In this and other areas of the African continent, cattle dung is often applied as a traditional remedy to the cut umbilical cord (neonatal tetanus, elsewhere unheard of, is by no means uncommon here); and the external genital organs of the women who deliver often have been previously mutilated by ritualistic clitoridectomy—the so-called "female circumcision."

In most of the world, it is the local midwives that comfort the woman in travail, and help her through the difficult pass. It is well that this be so, because the experience of all international health organizations has conclusively shown that no plan of public health will succeed, regardless of how well thought out, if it does not respect the local traditions dear to the people. Clearly, the prospects for improvement depend on educating the midwives, who, in the most destitute areas of the world, are illiterate and lack the most elementary notions of hygiene. But the problems that arise in this connection, formidable as the Gorgon and multiform as Proteus, have nothing to do with advanced biomedical technology. Their discussion does not belong here.

The Flowers of Evil in
the Garden of Biology

ONSIDER A MAN'S BEGINNINGS. BEFORE HIS FATHER AND mother are joined in sexual embrace, he is nothing: he does not exist. He has never been, throughout the eternity prior to that moment. Never. But this thought, that a whole infinity had to pass before he was rescued from naught, scarcely troubles him. What he is apprehensive about, if not terrified, is death. Most of us are, to some extent. Presumably, our fear arises from the awareness that we are to return to the nothingness whence we came. What troubles us is the going there, not the coming therefrom.

Why would it be that non-existence weighs more upon our hearts when regarded as future, than when evoked as past? It can only be because life is unidirectional, and we, who are immersed in its current, feel for what lies ahead only, not for what is left behind. We are creatures of the vital flow, which runs forward without pause, remitment, or reversal. Were it not so, we would feel appeased by considering the two immensities as equivalent: the infinite time that ran its course before my birth, and the eternity that shall flow after my death. Sad consolation: to try to soothe ourselves of the infinite time after death, with the thought of the infinite time before birth!

And yet, theoretically, we must admit that the equivalence is perfect. As Schopenhauer pompously put it, "the infinity *a parte post* without me cannot be any more fearful than the infinity *a parte ante* without me,"[1] the reason being that the two infinities are absolutely identical. If they seem distinct, he said, it is only because of the interposition of "an ephemeral life dream." May be. But to most men and women the Schopenhauerian calculation is a perfectly useless arithmetic. For in the human perspective there is no equivalence: life—this fleeting, precarious, insubstantial "dream"—weighs for us more than the combined sum of the two eternities, *ante* and *post*. If they do not bring themselves to believe this all the time, men and women succeed very well in believing it part of the time: at least during that brief interval when they join each other in a sexual embrace. For, make no mistake, they will embrace, and they will unite, and they will procreate. They have done so for millions of years; and although technology has in various ways modified procreation, there is reasonable assurance that it will not abolish these ancient practices any time soon.

Why are we brought into the world? Strange to tell, it is always because of someone else's motivation. A woman wishes to become a loving mother. A man wishes to satisfy his ego. Or both hatch the obscure, unspoken yearning to vicariously relive a life that neither one can restart over. It may also be that we come into the world unbidden, without anyone having requested our presence. It is then that we speak of our birth as "an accident,"—acknowledging, for once, the very large role that contingency plays in our lives. Here is the ultimate irony: to be rescued from nothingness thanks to someone else's carelessness.

If it were possible to ask us, it may well be that we would politely decline: "No, thank you, sir. And you too, madam. I truly appreciate your parental good will, but I really don't care to be born." But no one asks us. If haply we chance to elaborate a negative assessment of the circumstance of our birth, it will be always in retrospect that we conclude it was not worth it. Some unhappy souls may agree with Crates (365-285 B.C.), the ancient Cynic philosopher, when he said:

> "Why would anyone wish to tread the road of life? Wherever you turn, you shall descry all manner of ills. The courts resound with litigations. The home's solicitude is but a heavy cross. On firm land, harsh labor exhausts you; at sea, a thousand dangers oppress you. If you live long and are well off, your life courses in fear and anxious insecurity; but if poor, how hard is a life of indigence! Are you married? Plenty of cares come from that state. But if you are single, a life of solitude awaits you. Have children, and discover how hard it is to bring them up. Have none, and live like an orphan in the world. Are you young? Unstable, rash and voluble is youth; but old age is drained, feeble, and infirm. What remains, then, if any sanity resides in you, is to opt for either of these two extremes: never to have come out of the dank and narrow maternal enclosure, or, having come out, immediately to go dive in the unseen tenebrosity of the Styx."[2]

Optimum non nasci, "the best is not to be born" was the recommendation of Crates and some of his fellow pessimists in classical antiquity. Yes, but who among us ever had that luck? The most that can be said is that some people honestly believed in the philosophy behind the adage. Thus, Herodotus says of the Trausi, inhabitants of a region neighboring Thrace, that they mourned the birth of a baby. Friends and relatives gathered around the cradle to lament and to weep at the evocation of the sorrows that awaited the newly born on the road of life. In appropriate contrast, the Trausi custom was to celebrate with feasts and good cheer the death of one of their number.[3]

Thus, we are brought into existence, bodied forth, by forces that we cannot control. Interestingly, we are shaped gradually. Our being is granted us little by little, and it is not clear—not clear to me, anyway, although others are quite dogmatic—precisely when can we be called human beings. A stone is fully a stone from the start; a plant, as soon as the seed germinates, becomes a plant wholly: all in one piece. Many things acquire their being *d'emblée*. Not human beings. We are perpetually changing. As physical entities first, and later in our psychological persona; for even after we are fully formed we can still elect becoming this or that.

There lies before us an uncertain future, ceaselessly unfolding its long trail of indefiniteness. To live is to travel down this pathway of indecision, forced at every turn to make choices. It is up to us to choose this or that, but choose we must; for even when we decide to do nothing, that is also a choice. Which is why the existentialists said that human beings are "condemned to be free." However, the changes of our physical being take place at first by the compulsion of biological forces only. Early on, we are not expected to choose. Is it perhaps because we are not yet fully human?

Consider these beginnings. The maternal egg-cell, just penetrated by the sperm-cell, is stirred into a series of divisions. It cleaves into two "daughter cells," each of which divides into two, and each of these, in turn, into two, . . . and so on. The resulting cells crowd in a tight mass, that resembles nothing so much as a microscopic mulberry. It is the *morula*. At first, all the cells of the morula are alike, there is no differentiation or organization of any kind: there is no right or left side, no top and no bottom. Can we be called human beings at this point? It seems unlikely. Fluid begins to accumulate in the center of the mass of cells. And perhaps the future human being is never as close to perfection as while in this pristine, undifferentiated state, when it is spheroidal. The ancient Greeks recognized in the sphere the most perfect of shapes, for it can turn without requiring any space outside it. Xenophanes linked it to the divinity, since its starting point can be assumed to be at any place, and is thus perfect or "complete" Heraclitus acknowledged roundness as the supreme quality, for in it "beginning and end are common."[4]

Until then, the size of the developing being has scarcely changed. The fertilized egg—cell is cleft in two cells, then in four, then in eight, and so on, giving rise to ever smaller daughter cells, without increasing its total volume. The egg-cell is simply cut into many tiny pieces. When sixty four cells are formed, not only do they continue dividing, but now with each division they increase in size. Before that, the embryo took all the energy necessary for sustaining life from the maternal reserves that were offered it. Thereafter, it will become necessary to actively draw nourishment from the surrounding tissues.

The substances that it absorbs, it must transform into "human substance." Or, more properly speaking, into "individual human substance," as Jean Rostand wrote, since the embryo has to manufacture its own substance, "a particular protoplasm, a personal protoplasm, which is neither quite like its father's, nor quite like its mother's, but strictly its own: a protoplasm that will have nowhere its copy, and whereof it alone holds the secret."[5] Is this, then, the time for officially acknowledging the arrival of a new *individual* human being, albeit a microscopic one that looks like the fruit of the mulberry tree? On the face of it, it seems very doubtful. Moreover, most of the cells in this mass are destined to become placenta and associated structures. In some cases, as pathology teaches us, this is all that will be formed: embryo-supporting tissues, but no human embryo at all.

Then, a week after the initial generative act, or in the 6th to 7th post-coital day, as is said in technical parlance, the mass of cells has formed a millimeter-sized, fluid-filled vesicle, barely visible to the naked eye, called the *blastocyst*, and composed of 107 to 256 cells. It is no longer geometrically perfect, but somewhat flattened, and about the size of a pin's head. A mass of cells in its interior constitutes the human "bud," *i.e.*, the first rudiment of the embryo proper; the rest will form the placenta and supporting structures. Soon the inner mass of cells becomes discoidal (embryonic disk), and formed of superposed layers of cells: one that faces the outside, or *ectoderm,* and one internal, the *endoderm.* A third one, the *mesoderm,* is later interposed betweeen the two. Then, to the unbounded admiration and astonishment of anyone who cares to observe the subsequent development, this mass of cells undergoes a series of transfomations, far more spectacular than the celebrated metamorphoses of the developing butterfly.

About the eighteenth day, a furrow appears on the embryonic disk, marking its central axis that runs from its anterior to its posterior extremity. It is the early sketch of the central nervous system, whose anterior extremity swells to make the brain. At four weeks, the embryo is still less than three millimeters in length. It is very roughly sketched. Is this the first moment of the human condition? One would never suspect it. There is very little, in its external appearance, that evokes the human form: it is a bizarre animalcule. It has no arms or legs to speak of. If this is a human being, then in the beginning we are like *apodes*, degenerate fishes, eels or morays, limbless and finless. In the future neck region, transversal fissures appear— the *branchial* clefts—that are very much like the gills of fish. The heart has formed, but it is a straight tube; and it has begun to beat softly, propelling a rudimentary circulation that resembles, it too, that of some fishes.

All who have looked into this remarkable process never cease to be amazed. During embryonic development, the structure of the human being strikingly resembles that of lower animal forms. Karl Ernst von Baer (1792-1876) could write in 1821 that he kept, inside alcohol bottles, "two little embryos whose labels I failed to write, and later found it impossible to tell which class they belong to. They may be lizards, or little birds, or very early mammalians, so great is the similarity in the manner of formation of the head and trunk in these animals."[6] Thus, in embryonic life, the human

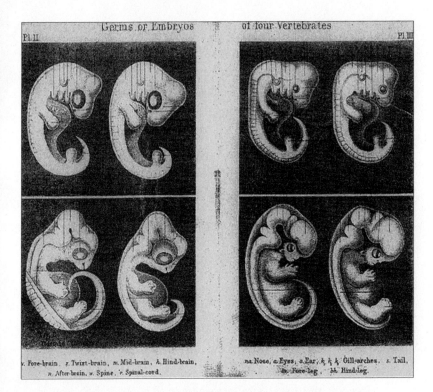

Germs or Embryos of four Vertebrates

Pl.II ... Pl.III

v. Fore-brain. *z.* Twixt-brain. *m.* Mid-brain. *h.* Hind-brain, *n.* After-brain. *w.* Spine. *r.* Spinal-cord.

na. Nose, *a.* Eyes, *o.* Ear, *k* *k* *k.* Gill-arches. *s.* Tail, *fe.* Fore-leg . *bh.* Hind-leg.

Comparison of embryos of different species. On plate II, left side of illustration, are shown: tortoise at 4th week (upper) and 6th week (lower), and chick at 4 (upper) and 8 days (lower). On plate III, right side of illustrations: dog at 4 weeks (upper) and at 6 weeks. Man is shown at the extreme right, at 4 weeks (upper) and 8 weeks (lower). Haeckel wished to emphasize the striking morphologic similarity across species. (*After Haeckel*)

being successively exhibits features that belong to protozoa, to annelids, to fishes, to reptiles, to batracians, and lastly to mammalians. It was inevitable that biologists would feel prompted to formulate a rational explanation of this process.

If human development exhibits transient resemblances to lower animal forms, said the evolutionists, it is because mankind evolved from primitive animals. Man "re-climbs his genealogic tree" every time he is formed inside his mother's womb. In the span of nine months, and in the enclosure of the maternal body, man travels backward the millenarian journey of evolution, and *is* successively single-celled organism, fish, reptile, batrachian, and so on. (If so, when, oh when, can he be declared unmistakably human?) It was the German physiologist Ernst Haeckel (1834-1919) who came up with the well known, canonic formula: "ontogenesis recapitulates phylogenesis." In other words, man's early embryonic development is an abridged version of the evolution of the human species, the memory of which has been preserved somehow, by the puissance of our genetics.

This was a striking idea, and although it was neither entirely due to Haeckel, nor, in the end, entirely correct (at no time is a young mammalian a fish), nonetheless it influenced profoundly our manner of thinking about embryology.

Despite the great similarities that may exist between a reptile, a bird, and a mammalian at early stages of embryonic development, Darwin had declared in 1842 that it is not true that during ontogenesis one passes through inferior animal forms.[7] But the idea of a "recapitulation" of phylogenesis has something in it that is uniquely intriguing. It continued to seize the imagination of biologists for many years, and up to our day, as is apparent in a recent learned treatise devoted to this topic by the brilliant scientist and writer Stephen Jay Gould.[8] Its impact was especially marked in comparative embryology, as it became clear that similarities between larvae or embryos of different species revealed unsuspected relationships useful for classification.

However, nineteenth century biologists abused Haeckel's concept of "recapitulation." Excessive use is commonly the fate of colorful ideas that have a strong appeal to the mind. Scientists imagined they saw in every minute embryonic structure the very features of precursor animal species, and this abusive interpretation ended up detracting from the real usefulness of the central idea. But, be that as it may, the fact cannot be ignored that developing human embryos exhibit transient structures that are like those of adult animals placed lower in the evolutionary scale. And what can this mean, if not that we are kith and kin of these other animal species, a fact otherwise confirmed by the modern tools of molecular genetics?

All of which sends us back to the question of what it means to be human, and whether there is a specific time in our formation when we may be said to have acquired the full human condition, the defining quality of a human being. Some say our being is not delivered to us gradually, but instantaneously, at conception. Conception is the beginning of the beginning: a moment before, the human being did not exist; a moment later, it *is*—irrevocably and with all the essential characteristics that define the human being. The seriousness with which this conclusion is urged became clear to me when, as a newly arrived immigrant in the United States, close to forty years ago, I worked as an intern in a Catholic hospital run by nuns.

I was assigned to the pathology laboratory, and every afternoon it was my duty to describe the specimens that had been removed at surgery, and submitted to the laboratory. The tissues came, as is customary, suspended in formalin fixative solution in adequately labeled, tightly capped bottles. As the evening approached I took out the specimens, dictated their description into an automatic tape recorder, and made tissue slices adequate for later microscopic examination; all according to a daily routine that is utterly familiar to anyone who has seen the work of a pathology laboratory.

The hospital was located in a mountainous region, in a beautiful setting. Through a window I could see the sky, usually blue when I started my routine, but turning crimson and gold before I finished, as the sun left the world to sink behind the mountains. Below, a spire and part of ivy-mantled walls was all I could see of a church; and behind it, a glimmering landscape, thick with rugged elms, slowly faded from me to be enfolded in shade, while I went on with my descriptions. It was not an unpleasant place to work in, considering the dreary, uncheerful listlessness that the popular sentiment attaches to hospitals.

Further to enliven the scene, a technician often turned on a portable radio, at low volume so as not to interfere with my dictation, but not so low that I could not tell what was playing. I have recollections of agitating a bottle with swirling fragments of prostatic tissue, to the strains of "Smoke Gets in Your Eyes," and laying out an inflamed appendix on the examining table, with the then fashionable "Fever" sung by Peggy Lee, in the background.

Inside short, wide flasks, we used to receive the fragments of tissue scraped off from the womb at surgery, during the procedure known familiarly as "D & C" for "dilatation and curettage." This operation, as the name clearly says, consists in the mechanical dilatation of the womb's entrance opening (the *os* of the uterine cervix) by introducing progressively wider metallic dilators, then scraping off the inner lining of the uterus with a curette. This is needed to stop the bleeding after an incomplete abortion, in which retained, ill attached fragments of placental tissue are the cause of copious, some times life-jeopardizing hemorrhage. The abortion can be spontaneous or criminally induced: the treatment of the bleeding is the same. It goes without saying that the identical procedure is used to perform an abortion in a normal non-bleeding pregnant woman. However, in a Catholic hospital this would not have been permitted. Accordingly, the specimens that I saw were always labeled "incomplete *spontaneous* abortion."

I was instructed to leave the description of the fragments of tissue retrieved by "D & C" to the end. I soon understood why. Late in my workday, a solemn ambiance waxed instantaneously in the room. The technician quickly turned off the radio, and everyone did his or her best to appear busy. A humorless, somewhat grim-faced supervisor—nun in charge of our area had appeared. She came by my work bench, where I had carefully set aside all the appropriate bottles. Then, placed in front of the row of flasks, rosary in hand, eyes downcast, she said a few prayers, made the sign of the cross and sprinkled holy water on the bottles, while the rest of us looked quiet and contrite. I used to stand to one side with my head lowered, unable to resume my work until the ritual finished.

What did she petition for in her prayers? I never could tell. Surely not, as in the poet's line, for "obedient passions and a will resigned." Perhaps for love and forgiveness. What is certain is that the ceremony was performed because of the possibility that a human embryo might be somewhere inside those bottles, among those tissues; a rudimentary human being, endowed, nonetheless, with an immortal soul. Therefore it behooved the faithful to implore the mercy of heaven for its benefit. The ancients believed that the body was not "animated," that is, did not receive the soul (Latin *anima*) that vivified it, until the fortieth day of gestation in males, or on day eighty or ninety in females.

The Catholic Church always maintained, contrary to some oriental religions, that human souls do not exist independently of bodies, and do not antedate them, but that the soul is divinely imbued into a previously formed body. An obstetrician-*philosophe*, such as the Enlightenment produced, reminded his contemporaries in a textbook[9] that this is how the Almighty proceeded with the first man, since it is set down in *Genesis* (chapter 2, 7) that the Lord formed Adam out of the loam of the earth, then "breathed into his nostrils the breath of life." So it is, presumably, with his descendants: human beings are first created from seeds—male and female—and after their formation the Lord blows upon them the vital breath.

But what is the precise timing of the divine insufflation? The question is dealt with in a book of most remarkable title: *Sacred Embryology*,[10] written by reverend Cangiamila, priest and inquisitor of Palermo, and published in 1745. The author tells us that, following Plato, Protagoras, and other ancient worthies, a medical authority of Prague named Johannes Marcus had proposed that the soul enters the fetus at birth, with the first breath. But this could not be, because Holy

Scripture recorded that St. John the Baptist had leaped inside his mother's abdomen at six months of gestation; therefore he was already "animated" at that early age. On the authority of St. Basil and others, it was best to make no distinctions between animate and inanimate fetuses: this is a very hard determination to make in many cases. Animate versus inanimate? Since it was difficult to tell one from the other, the priest should not deny the Church sacraments to any.

This was the central problem. Cangiamila quotes a book by Girolamo Fiorentini, entitled "On Doubtful Men, or the Baptism of Abortions," published in 1658, with unconditional approval of the theological authorities of Prague, Vienna, Paris, and Salamanca. In that treatise, the question was squarely posed: What should a priest do when called to the bedside of a woman who has miscarried, or aborted, or delivered an unviable fetus? Considering that the time of "animation" is doubtful, and that it could be since conception, a priest was under obligation to baptize "the germ of a man, even if it is no bigger than a grain of barley"; even when still ill formed and indistinct (just like those irregular, bloody fragments of nondescript tissue obtained from a "D & C," which I used to handle every afternoon); or, if more or less formed, even if it shows no evidence of movement or any other signs of life, since it is well known that bodily movement may be absent while the blood still stirs. About the only condition that justifies withholding baptism is advanced putrefaction—all other signs of death may be deceiving. But, adds Cangiamila, baptism must then be conditional. First, because the priest does not know whether his subject is dead or alive; and secondly, because the baptismal water may not reach it, since it may be hidden behind membranes and protected by amniotic fluid.

It seems that, before the mentioned treatise, no one had proposed the need to baptize *all* the embryos and fetuses. The Roman ritual had not envisaged the baptism of abortions, and the author proposed a new formula. He advanced a prudent disclaimer: he did not wish to impose a new rite, but only to set forth the reasons that could engage priests to adopt it. The proposed formula of conditional baptism says: "If you are apt to receive baptism . . .", or "If you are actually alive . . .", or "If unbaptized . . . I baptize you" (*Si tu es capax baptismi* . . . , or *Si vivis* . . . , or *Si non es baptisatus* . . . *ego te baptiso*). Was any of these the formula pronounced by the nun of my recollection? I could not tell. But I found it remarkable that someone should worry over the transcendent destiny of a human embryo. I somehow felt then, and still feel today, that a hieratic, reverential or solemn attitude, is due to the "rudiment" of man.

No one writes textbooks entitled "Sacred Embryology" any more. Today, we are apt to hear of Descriptive Embryology, Experimental Embryology, and—most of all—Molecular Embryology. The de-sacralization of embryology is almost complete: the composition of the entire human genome has been exposed, and we are told that our developmental fate lies not in the hands of Divine Providence, as Pascal would have us believe, but in our genetic constitution. A form of fatalism is replaced by another, "scientific fatalism."

However, human beings have a fundamental need to experience the preternatural: an almost physiological need to be affected by the charm, the mystery and majesty of superior forces, vaster than any that human intelligence can apprehend. As Mircea Eliade[11] has pointed out, even the most profane and avowedly non-religious materialist lives, often without realizing it, of mythico-religious beliefs and practices. Man needs periodically to plunge into the noumenal; hankers for experience of the transcendent; yearns to find an opening to another dimension, different and conceived as higher than that of the purely material world that surrounds him. To casually disregard this yearning, or to lay it at the door of simple ignorance, would be to deny a specifically human attribute. This is why the de-sacralization of Nature can never be total, cannot be carried to an extreme.

The religious mind sees in the structure of the world the manifestation of the sacred in its various modalities. I would suggest that this revelation—this hierophany—nowhere comes through with greater force than in the process of embryonic development, which is compendium and paradigm of all the possibilities of existence. Nor is there any need for mystico-religious references: the process of embryonic development is, without exaggeration, miraculous. That a microscopic cell should begin dividing, and the resulting parts aggregating, folding, moving, and rearranging, until it forms a human being, is a phenomenon far beyond words. A greater portent can scarcely be imagined. Ovid, in all his outlandish *Metamorphoses*, did not describe a more incredible, bizarre phenomenon. For the transformation of Daphne into a laurel tree, or Lycaon into a wolf, or Io into a cow, seem less far-fetched occurrences, less fantastic, than a viscid microscopic globule ceaselessly splitting itself, and undergoing exquisitely coordinated changes that make it resemble an amorphous mass, then a mulberry, a hollow ball, a trilayered disk, and then successively a worm, a tadpole, a fish, a mammal . . . finally becoming a real human being. All in nine months! That is all it takes to produce a being fully equipped to become, given the opportunity to mature, a sensitive and rational being, with thoughts, passions, emotions, spirituality, religion and science.

Think of this: a gooey mass of molecules that, in a short time, becomes a being possessed of the ability to explain how a gooey mass of molecules can become a rational being. This is the enigma of enigmas, the central problem for biology for all time, to my eye the most important scientific mystery. More compelling than the exploration of outer space or the investigation of the intimate structure of matter, because it touches us more immediately.

Scientific understanding of embryonic development achieved astounding progress in the last few decades. This advance was fostered by our ability to manipulate DNA, and therefore the genes, since genes are made up of this molecule. Genes are now identified, isolated, reproduced in as many copies as desired, and their composition—their "anatomy"—described in minute detail. The filamentous structure of DNA can be cut at specific points chosen at will; the cut may be repaired; the loose ends may be spliced together; or fragments of other DNA segments inserted between the cuts. All this is remarkable. It means the power to tinker with the immense quantities of DNA of complex organisms. By virtue of this ability, instead of asking what is the composition of a living being, as formerly, scientists ask how is a living being, animal or plant, put together. The question of how is a fruit fly (*Drosophila*) or a worm (*C. elegans*) assembled, is already largely elucidated; the building of other, more complex organisms is now being studied. The next step is intervention upon mankind.

Hence the distrust of biology. This is a new phenomenon. Until now, if science ever inspired any diffidence in the public, it was against physics and chemistry, because these sciences gave us, together with remarkable benefits, the distinct possibility of being obliterated from the world in a single, apocalyptic conflagration. Biology had escaped any such blame. After all, it stood in a lower rung of the hierarchy of knowledge. It did not have the prestige that comes with exact calculation and unerring prediction. Moreover, the biologic sciences were the sustaining pillars of medicine, and therefore eminently atruistic in orientation. They were allies in the fight against pain and suffering; they were helping us to suppress illness.

But, lo and behold! In the last half-century it is biology that begins to be perceived negatively. For it begins to be able to control human behavior with psychotropic drugs; and its doings are associated to the world's overpopulation; and it threatens to dislocate the traditional roles of the family; and there is even talk of cloning human individuals, raising the specter of thousands of human beings copied and reproduced mechanically, like so many robots. But the idea of performing in the laboratory experiments that do not occur spontaneously in Nature, carries even greater terror. That genes from one animal can be cut, removed, inserted in another living being, and made to function, sometimes across barrier species (the firefly's genes, for instance, have been grafted unto plants, obtaining plants that glow; likewise, luminiscence genes from the jellyfish *Aequerea victoria* inserted into the genome of mice, give rise to mice that fluoresce with a green shine),[12] is something that we find deeply disturbing. It is an achievement that calls to mind images of monsters and fantastic beings, like those imagined by the fifteenth century painter Hieronymus Bosch: men with fish head, or with a pig's snout and a serpent for a tail—nightmarish hybrids with which Bosch wished to represent human folly and sin, but which appear to have become a hallucinating, shocking reality.

In the formerly pleasant, restful garden of biology, and more precisely in biomedicine, evil flowers appear to have suddenly sprung. And the air fills with the enervating, musty aroma of decay that emanates from them. Truth to tell, no flower is "evil," much in spite of Baudelaire's famous poem. But according as to how they are used, the most beautiful may lose their charm and become deadly. The flowers of the nightshade plant are a pretty sight; its shiny dark berries invite a taste; and yet, children who eat them immoderately die poisoned. Just so the unwise use of the flowers of biomedicine, so prevalent in human reproduction, often end up transforming a beauteous parterre into Lucifer's garden.

A Troubling Bouquet

· The mandragora in the garden, because the oldest and most often used, is In Vitro Fertilization (IVF). It consists in putting the male's sperm and the female's egg-cell in contact with each other, but outside the woman's body, in a plastic dish (not a test tube, as some erroneously assume); the resulting embryo is put back into the woman's womb, where it develops to term. Conception is therefore de-sexualized: henceforward it becomes a matter for laboratorians, not lovers.

Although the first baby so conceived was born on July 25, 1978, preparatory work antedated the birth for many years. So did opposition: irate headlines had thundered against it clamoring "Ban the Test-Tube Baby" (*Sun*, February 25, 1970), and dubbing it "Test-Tube Stud Farming" (*Sunday Express*, March 1st, 1970). Staid ecclesiastics and renowned scientists condemned the procedure. Some equated it to infanticide, since during IVF some embryos had to be destroyed. Be that as it may, one has to admit that making conception possible without sex was eminently newsworthy. Which is why the first woman made pregnant via this technic, a British subject, was literally assailed by journalists. The clinic where she was going to deliver was invaded by reporters disguised as janitors, boiler makers, or nurses. The *paparazzi* intrusiveness was carried to new heights when one of them triggered a false bomb alarm that required evacuation of all patients, not excepted those just subjected to surgery, from the building.

Today, IVF is routine. It is estimated that at least 300,000 children were thus conceived. But what will happen to them no one knows. For just about now they are beginning to reach the age at which they could reproduce, and it is a question whether their progeny will be normal. Mark that IVF itself is not innocuous. More than one embryo is usually implanted, because every clinic strives to show excellent rates of successful implantation, and the more embryos placed in the womb, the higher the chances of a "take." Yet, multiple pregnancies are risky for mother and children. That one is prone to serious complications, such as thrombosis and embolism, or the development of diabetes. The babies suffer most grievously from the effects of prematurity, since their gestation is usually shorter than normal. Neonatal brain damage and lung diseases may leave them with life-long disabilities.

Drugs that stimulate ovulation are widely used in the treatment of infertility. They are so effective, that they can be blamed for the increase in multiple pregnancies that is observed throughout the world. During fifty years our planet saw less than fifty sets of quadruplets. Today, this number is matched or exceeded in a single year. Multiple births have increased six-fold in twenty-five years.[13] And the magnitude of the multiple gestations borders on the grotesque.

A few years ago, a couple from Albany, New York, Michelle and Norman Haner, attracted attention when the woman delivered septuplets. Soon they were matched by Bobbi and Kenny McCaughey, of Iowa, who emulated them on November of 1997, but only to be surpassed by Nkem Chukwu, a 27 year-old Nigerian immigrant, who—exceeding all the predictions of the ancients and most modern authors about the number of fetuses that may be housed simultaneously in the maternal womb—gave birth to octuplets in 1998. The smallest of her babies, a girl, weighed a mere 320 grams (10.3 oz.) and fit in the palm of an adult's hand. She was born twelve days before the other seven, and died after a few days of extrauterine existence. Because they were thirteen weeks premature, they suffered a number of very dangerous complications. They were treated in the Texas Children's Hospital of Houston, which boasts one of the largest and most sophisticated neonatal intensive care units in the world, at the cost of two million dollars. Two had eye surgery, and were kept alive by highly complex, technically advanced medical instruments. Nevertheless, the media extolled these births, glorifying them as meritorious record-breaking prowess.

The media generally rhapsodize about the "miracles" wrought by reproductive biomedicine. Indeed, since the fundamental premiss is that life is a God-given, precious gift, it follows that the more of it, the better. The McCaugheys, parents of septuplets, wrote a book appropriately entitled "Seven From Heaven," and the Nigerian parents of the Houston octuplets declared in a television interview of December 22, 1998, that they were "very excited and grateful to God." When asked whether she intended to have more babies, the mother replied ". . . if God does it, we won't call it an accident."[14] Clearly, the minute one invokes the intervention of Divine Providence, any hope for a fruitful discussion of the perils and limitations of reproductive medicine is annulled *ipso facto*.

A reporter (Diane Sawyer) who interviewed the mother, gave free course to the kind of maternal sentimentalism that tends equally to abrogate any expression of concern for the ill advised practices of reproductive biomedicine. Said she: ". . . It is one thing to have a debate about fertility medicine, quite another to feel the warmth of a tiny touch. The questions seem to vanish with that first smile."[15]

The questions that so swiftly vanish are many, indeed: questions about the life-long handicaps of prematurity, which include learning disabilities, impaired respiratory function, and many others; questions about the many parents who, not qualifying for fame and television appearances (quadruplets today make no news), are left to struggle alone with tremendous physical and financial burdens; questions about the dangers to health that the mother is made to undergo during multiple gestation; or about the millions of uninsured, premature babies who need expensive neonatal hospital care, but must do without, while valuable resources are derived to sensational, publicity-attracting cases.

"Evil flowers" is probably a bad simile; their luxuriance rather likens them to weeds. If technology causes problems, more technology is the remedy. If too many fetuses are present in the womb, there is always "selective reduction," a fine euphemism for killing one or more. This can be done with a lethal injection guided by ultrasound. But this procedure, alas, is not without risk. The mother may feel guilt, and fall into a depression. Or the "reduction" is not as "selective"as intended, and all fetuses are miscarried.

Is infertility due to too few spermatozoa, or to their decreased motility? Not to worry. If sperm acts shy when it approaches the ovum, it can always be encouraged. A single sperm-cell can be picked up with a pointed pipette, and directly injected into the egg-cell, thereby circumventing any male shyness. This wild flower (still not as common as a weed) goes by the name of "intracytoplasmic sperm injection," or ICSI. The suspicion is afoot, however, that children conceived by this method may be subject to more chromosomal anomalies and malformations than those brought into existence in the conventional way. Even if they are normal, the boys could inherit the decreased sperm motility of their father. Of course, in that case, they, too, will have ICSI.

If the problem of sperm or egg-cell is beyond our not inconsiderable present means, we can always use someone else's gametes. They are for sale. Entrepreneurs have de-mystified the "procreative potency" of the ancients, and turned it into a commercial product. Fear not a debasement of the race. Today, sperm donors are recruited among the *élite*. University students read advertisements in their very *alma mater* magazines that say: "Pay tuition with sperm (or eggs)." A sperm donor is paid between $35 and $50 dollars per "delivery," and may give up to three "deliveries" per week. Egg donors get more money, but the procedure to collect egg-cells is no bargain; why, when you take into account that there must be injections of hormones that stimulate ovulation (and in the process may cause ovarian cysts, hemorrhage, and perhaps predispose to cancer), and that the harvesting requires a laparoscopic operation, it is no wonder some women donors conclude that a few thousand dollars are "not worth it."

It goes without saying that harvesting sperm-cells is safe, and a business man, Robert K. Graham, in 1980 founded the Repository for Germinal Choice, a firm committed to sell the sperm of "outstandingly intelligent and healthy men," including Nobel Prize laureates. At least one of these, William Shockley, inventor of the transistor, contributed to the repository. This bold eugenic effort, however, has thus far not produced a noteworthy leader of mankind.

But what about all the bother and inconvenience of these procedures? In her truly excellent book, *The Clone Age*, Lori B. Andrews mentions plans of the Xytex Corporation to sell franchises to drugstores.[16] Presumably, the company would install a liquid nitrogen tank in the drugstore, to keep the sperm vials frozen. For every vial sold, the company would pay a certain amount to the vendor. There is money to be made here, since the proportion of women who suffer from thinking themselves infertile is high. Thus, ladies could pick up in their neighborhood drugstore, together with cosmetics, vitamins and aspirin, a vial of semen that they could later insert into themselves at home, for it is not unwarranted to think that the sellers would soon be promoting kits with special applicators (a rubber bulb, a writer noted, as used in the kitchen for basting, would do).

The problems with donated semen are not few. The sooner it is frozen, the better for its freshness; but testing for hereditary and infectious diseases may take time, and it is impractical to test for every possible contaminant. Donors are checked, but some diseases are not immediately apparent. So it is that one donor transmitted polycystic kidney disease to an undefined number of children conceived with his sperm. Apparently he had donated 320 vials before it was discovered that he had an inheritable condition and was taken off the donor list.

Another noted case was that of the infamous Dr. Cecil Jacobson, a renowned physician with a solid background in reproductive medicine, who used his own semen to inseminate his patients, without informing them. Yet one more mishap was described by Lori B. Andrews[17] in her fascinating book. A technician, after completing an ICSI procedure, unwittingly fertilized a second maternal gamete when he used an imperfectly cleaned pipette that still contained a single spermatozoon from another donor. The mother ended up having twins, each one of a different race.

Post-menopausal pregnancies are the henbane in Lucifer's garden. When a sixty-two year old grandmother is made to become pregnant thanks to IVF and heavy hormonal treatment, and thus enabled to gestate the fetuses conceived with her daughter's egg-cell and her son-in-law's sperm, there is an outburst of media cooing and jubilation. The older woman gave "the gift of life" that her daughter so ardently desired but could not produce herself. She is a paragon of motherly love and generosity. But amidst the plaudits and felicitations, no one asks if it is good medicine to subject a post-menopausal grandmother to the very real dangers of multiple pregnancy. No one stops to ponder that this heroic, generous lady will be both mother and grandmother to the children. Therefore, she becomes something like sister of her daughter (who herself will be both mother and aunt to her children) and wife of her son-in-law. The lines of filiation, the family links and relations as we understand them, and as we have understood them for millennia, are suddenly scrambled, irretrievably entangled by the "miracle" of reproductive medicine.

What I have called flowers of evil, others might name absurdities, transgressions, misdeeds, rashness, or thoughtlessness. They proliferate because almost any new idea, as soon as it appears, is legitimated by the media and transformed into action. This is done largely because of hubris, the quintessentially human foible; because of an intimate conviction that knowledge leads to technology, which permits to improve the existing conditions; and because of a blind belief that "everything is knowable and everything is improvable," as the Cartesians maintained.

Perhaps it is time to re-examine these beliefs. In the famous opening of the second chapter of Descartes' *Discourse of the Method*, the philosopher takes flight comparing Nature and human industry. He asks us if it is not true that modern cities, traced by an architect with geometrical regularity, are better, more beautiful and agreeably proportioned than the disorderly spectacle of winding, narrow streets of ancient towns that grew without the benefit of urban planning. And I cannot help thinking that this literary period, however impressive it may have sounded in the seventeenth century, has lost its effectiveness to modern ears. For many urban dwellers, immersed in the chaos of today's polluted, impersonal cities, have plenty of reasons to prefer the quaint ancient village.

Somewhere in his thoughtful work, Paul Valéry describes an episode of his life that impresses me like an allegory of today's quandaries in reproductive medicine. He tells us that, during the second world war, the French forces had been rapidly overwhelmed by the advances of the German army. In great haste, before the enemy would be able to take over the equipment still in possession of the defeated French, the most valuable weapons were loaded onto a ship, and put to sea. Valéry was a passenger in this boat. In their precipitation, the fleeing men could not embark all the necessary navigation equipment. Shortly after reaching the open sea, a dense fog descended upon them, and covered them completely. The wind started blowing. And, for a time, they drifted aimlessly, in an ominous silence, tense, apprehensive, fearful of enemy submarines. And Valéry reflected on their situation: they were aboard an impressive warship, armed to the teeth with the most advanced weapons that the mind of man could conceive, and yet floating without bearings, at the mercy of the waves, not knowing what was going to happen to them.

Is this not like our own situation? We have at our disposal the most sophisticated scientific equipment that ever was. Molecular biology is now in a position to alter Nature. We fancy ourselves masters and possessors of the universe. For the first time in history, we have the means and the ability to modify ourselves. And we know not where we are going, or even where we should go.

Notes

To Begin at the Beginning . . . or Almost

1. Frederick von Schlegel: *The Philosophy of Life.* Lecture V. Translated from the German by A.J.W. Morrison. Henry G. Bohn, London, 1847. Page 77.

2. Max Delbrück: Evolution of Life, Chapter 2 in: *Mind from Matter? An Essay in Evolutionary Epistemology.* Blackwell Scientific Publications, Palo Alto. 1986. Page 32.

3. Nicolas Malebranche: *Eclaircissements sur La Recherche de la Vérité.* See:XV th *Eclaircissement* in: *Oeuvres.* (in two vols.) Vol. 1 Gallimard, Bibliothèque de la Pléiade. Paris. 1979.

4. C.F. von Weizsäcker: *The History of Nature.* University of Chicago Press, 1940. (First published as *Die Geschichte der Natur*, Hirzel Verlag, Zurich, Switzerland).

5. Bernice Wuethrich: Why sex? Putting the theory to the test. *Science* vol. 281, Number 5385, September 25, 1998 (an issue devoted to the evolution of sex). Pages 1980-1982.

6. Georges-Louis Leclerc, Count de Buffon : *Histoire Naturelle*, in: *Oeuvres de Buffon, Avec des Extraits de Dauberton.* Furne et Cie. Paris. 1837. See vol 3.

7. J. Rodolfo Wilcox: *Lo Stereoscopio dei Solitari.* 2nd edition. Adelphi. Milan. 1989. Pages 19-20.

8. The concept of a "Mitochondrial Eve" was first suggested by Allan Wilson, Rebecca Cann and Mark Stoneking, of the University of California, Berkeley, in an article entitled "Mitochondrial DNA and human evolution," which appeared in *Nature*, in January of 1987.

Related material may be found in the following: Templeton, A.R.: Human origins and analysis of mitochondrial DNA sequences. *Science*, vol. 255, 1992. Page 737.; Templeton, A.R.: The "Eve" hypothesis. A genetic critique and reanalysis. *American Antrhropologist*. Vol. 95, 1993. Pages 51-72; Wilson, A. C. and Cann, R.L.: The recent African genesis of humans. *Scientific American* (April 1992): pages 68-73.

9. Thomas De Quincey: Shakespeare. Chapter One in: *Biographical Essays*. Ticknor & Fields, Boston. 1861.

10. Weismann, August (Friedrich Leopold): *Die Kontinuität des Keimplasmas als Grudlage einer Theorie der Vererbung*. Gustav Fischer, Jena. 1885. After expounding on his theory of the "continuity of the germ plasm," Weismann also developed his ideas in a more comprehensive manner in his book, *Das Keimplasma: Eine Theorie der Vererbung*. Gustav Fischer, Jena. 1892. This work exists in English translation: *The Germ Plasm: A Theory of Heredity*. (Translated by N.N. Parker and H. Rönnfeld)t: Charles Scribners and Sons. New York. 1915.

11. Jean-Pierre Vernant: *Un, deux, trois: Eros*. Chapter 8 in: *L'Individu, La Mort, L'Amour. Soi-même et l'autre en Grèce ancienne*. Gallimard. Paris. 1989.

Believe Only the Delivery

1. Anatole France: *Rabelais*. Translated and with an introduction by Ernest Boyd. Henry Holt, New York. 1028, page 136.

2. The quotation is from "The Dream of Death," one of several "dreams" or halllucinating fantasies by Quevedo, literary genius and complex personality of senventeenth century Spain, who could write one minute a pious sermon full of erudite references to Holy Scripture, and the next minute a cynical, cruel satire of the customs and follies of his day. See: Francisco de Quevedo y Villegas: *El Sueño de la Muerte*, in: *Los Sueños*, edited by Ignacio Arellano. Cátedra, Letras Hispánicas. Madrid 1991, Pp. 387-368. (Author's translation).

3. The medieval tradition is consigned in a manuscript kept in the *Bibliothèque Nationale* of Paris, classified as B.N. # 1543. It was reproduced, accompanied by a philological study, in: Claude Thomasset: *Dialogue de Placides et Timéo*. Librairie Droz. Geneva. 1980.

4. Ambroise Paré: *Rapport des Filles. Si Elles Sont Vierges ou Non*. Chapter XLV in: *Textes Choisis*. Presented and commented by Louis Delaruelle and Marcel Sendrail. Société Les Belles Lettres. Paris, 1953. Pages 172-173.

5. Nicolas Venette: *La Génération de l'Homme, ou Tableau de l'Amour Conjugal Considéré dans l'État de Mariage.* Parme, 1696. (First edition published in 1685).

6. Auguste Debay: *La Vénus Féconde et Callipédique.* E. Dentu. Paris, 1881. Pp. 32-33.

7. Charles Mayo Goss (editor): *Anatomy of the Human Body by Henry Gray,* 29th edition. Lea & Febiger, Philadelphia, 1973.

8. See Giulia Sisa's essay, "The seal of virginity," in: Michel Feher, Ramona Nadaff, and Nadia Tazi (eds.): *Fragments for a History of the Human Body. Part Three.* Zone Books, New York, 1990. Pages 143-156. For further ideas of virginity in history, see also from Giulia Sisa: *Le Corps Virginal.* Vrin, Paris. 1987.

9. Quoted by Giula Sisa: *loc. cit.*

10. Peter Kandela: Egypt's trade in hymen repair. Lancet. Vol. 347; 1996, page 1615.

11. This information is supplied in one of the several communications published in the British Medical Journal in 1998, concerning the ethical implications of correcting the lacerations of the hymen consequent upon the initiation of sexual activity, in other words, the restoration of virginity. See: A. Logmans and collaborators, from the Daniel den Hoed Clinic, Rotterdam, Netherlands: "Should doctors reconstruct the vaginal introitus of adolescent girls to mimic the virginal state? Who wants the procedure and why." *BMJ* (British Medical Journal) Volume 316 (No.7219) 1998. Pages 459-60. See also, in the same volume, articles of the same title, subtitled "Surgery is not what it seems," by L. F. Ross, on page 462; and "Cultural complexities should not be ignored," by E. Webb, also page 462.

12. E. Girela, J.A. Lorente, J.C. Alvarez, M.D.Rodrigo, M. Lorente and W. Villanueva: Indisputable double paternity in dizygous twins. *Fertility & Sterility* Vol. 67; (number 6), June 1997. Pages 1159-1161.

13. On the paternity of Thomas Jefferson, as investigated by modern methods of DNA analysis, and the comments that this investigation elicited, see: E.A. Foster and collaborators: Jefferson fathered slave's last child [letter]. *Nature.* Vol. 396 (6706), November 5, 1998 pages 13-14. Correspondece and comments appeared in *Nature* Vol. 396 (6706), November 5, 1998, pages 27-28; and Vol.397 (6714), Jan 7, 1999, page 32. See also: E. Marshall: Which Jefferson was the father? [news section]. *Science,* Vol. 283 (5399): January 1999, pages 153-154.

14. Ronald G. Davidson: More genes for sale: The Iceland genomic story. *Annals of the Royal College of Physicians and Surgeons of*

Canada. Vol. 32 (Number 4), June 1999. Pages 208-210.

15. Anatole France's critique of Maupassant's *Pierre et Jean* was originally published in the Parisian periodical *Le Temps* on January 15, 1888. It is reproduced as an appendix in the edition of *Pierre et Jean* published in 1959 by Garnier Publishers, Paris, with introduction and notes of Pierre Cogny.

Saga of the Womb, or The Perils of the Mother

1. Mircea Eliade: *Shamanism. Archaic Technics of Ecstasy.* Princeton University Press, Bollingen Series LXXVI, 2nd printing, 1974. Page 37.

2. The comment is by Arthur Platt, translator in: J.A. Smith and W.D. Ross (editors) Aristotle's *Generation of Animals*, Volume 5 in the series The Works of Aristotle, Clarendon Press, Oxford, 1958 reprint of 1912 edition. All quotations from this work of Aristotle refer to this edition.

3. Sherwin B. Nuland: *The Wisdom of the Body.* Alfred A.Knopf, New York, 1997, page 171.

4. The symbolism of ornithomorphism is discussed by Mircea Eliade in *Shamanism,* pages 156-157 (See note 1, above).

5. Karl Sudhoff: *Ein Beitrag zur Geschichte der Anatomie im Mittelalter.* (Studies on the History of Medicine, Vol. 4). Barth, Leipzig, 1908, page 27 ff.

6. See Fridolf Kudlien: The Seven Cells of the uterus: the doctrine and its roots. *Bulletin of the History of Medicine*, Vol. 39; 1965. Pages 415-423.

7. Aelian: *On Animals.* Book XII, 16. Translated by A. L. Scholfield. In 3 vols. Loeb Classical Library. Harvard University Press, Cambridge. 1972. Vol. 3, Page 33.

8. Soranus: *Gynecology.* Translated by Owsei Temkin. Johns Hopkins University Press. Baltimore, 1991. See Book I, 10. Page 11.

9. Gaston Bachelard (1884-1962), distinguished French intellectual and poet, devoted several books to an exploration of the relationship between what is usually called poetical imagination, and the world of reality. Thus, in respective works he had much to say about imagination and fire, water, or space. The quotation is taken from a chapter devoted to "Maternal and Feminine Water" in: Gaston Bachelard: *L'Eau et les Rêves. Essai Sur l'Imagination de la Matière.* Librairie José Corti, Paris. 1942.

10. Mircea Eliade: *Images et Symboles. Essais sur le Symbolisme Magico-Religieux.* Gallimard, Paris. 1952 (reprinted in 1980). See Chapter 4, entitled *"Remarques sur le symbolisme des coquillages."*

11. G.S.Dawes: Breathing before birth in animals and man. *New England Journal of Medicine.* Vol. 290, 1974. Page 557.

12. A. Jost and A. Policard: *Contribution expérimentale à l'étude du développement du poumon chez le lapin. Archives d'Anatomie Microscopique* Vol. 37, 1948. Page 323. See also: Thomas Hansen and Anthony Corbet: "Lung Development and Function." Chapter 48 in: H. William Taeusch and Roberta Ballard (editors): *Avery's Diseases of the Newborn.* 7th Edition. W.B. Saunders, Philadelphia, 1998.

13. G. L. Streeter: Focal deficiencies in fetal tissues and their relationship to intrauterine amputations. *Contributions to Embryology of the Carnegie Institute.* Vol. 22, 1930. Pages 1-15.

14. Henry Ernest Sigerist: *Primitive and Archaic Medicine.* Vol. 1 of *A History of Medicine.* New York, 1951.

15. François de Rabelais: *Pantagruel,* Book Third. In: *The Portable Rabelais,* selected, translated and edited by Samuel Putnam. Viking, New York. 1946.

16. William Harvey: *The Works of William Harvey, M.D.* Translated by R. Willis. London, 1847. Page 542.

17. For a superb study of seventeenth century Dutch painting in its relation to the medical knowledge of the era, see: Laurinda S. Dixon: *Perilous Chastity, Women and Illness in Pre-Enlightenment Art and Medicine.* Cornell University Press, Ithaca. 1995.

18. Domenighetti G., Luraschi P., Marazzi A.: Hysterectomy and the sex of the gynecologist. *New England Journal of Medicine.* Vol. 313, 1985. Page 1942.

19. Gianfranco Domenighetti and Antoine Casabianca: Performing hysterectomy in low income women may be easier than educating them [letter, comment]. *BMJ (British Medical Journal)* Vol. 314 (No. 7091), May 10, 1997. Page 1417. See additional comments by the same authors in: Role of hysterectomy is lower among female doctors and lawyers' wives. *BMJ* Vol. 314 (No. 7075) January 18, 1997. Pages 160-161. Also R.J. Lilford: Hysterectomy: Will it pay the bills in 2007? *BMJ* Vol. 315 (No. 7108) . September 6, 1997. Page 603.

20. Kierulff K.H., Guzinski G.M., Langenberg P.W., Stolley P.D., Moye N.E., and Kazandjian A.: Hysterectomy and race. *Obstetrics & Gynecology.* Vo. 82 (no.5), November 1993. Pages 757-764.

21. Lepine L.A., Hillis S.D., Marchbanks P.A., Koonin L.M.,

Morrow B., Kieke B.A., and Wilcox L.S.: Hysterectomy surveillance—
United States, 1980-1993. *Morbidity and Mortality Weekly Report.
CDC Surveillance Summaries.* Volume 46 (No.4) August 8, 1997.
Pages 1-15.

On Female "Impressionism"

1. Lazzaro Spallanzani: *Expériences pour servir a l'histoire de la
génération des animaux et des plantes. Avec une ébauche de l'histoire
des êtres organisés avant leur fécondation, par Jean Senebier.* Pavie &
Paris, P.J. Duplain. 1787. See also the edition published by Lacombe,
Paris. 1769. An English translation is: *Dissertations Relative to the
Natural History of Animals and Vegetables.* J. Murray, London. 1789.

2. Clara Pinto-Correia: *The Ovary of Eve. Eggs and Sperm and
Preformation.* University of Chicago Press, 1997.

3. Carl Friedrich Burdach: *Traité de Physiologie.* (French translation from the German by A.J. L. Jourdan). In 9 vols. Paris, 1831-1841.
See vol. 1, pages 332-344.

4. Publius Vergili Maronis: *Bucolica et Georgica* (in Latin).
MacMillan & Co. London. 1965.

5. Pliny the Elder: *Natural History.* (In 10 vols.) 2nd edition.
Translated by H. Rackham. Vol. 3. Harvard University Press.
Cambridge. 1983. Pages 113-119.

6. Aristotle: *De Generatione Animalium.* Translated by Arthur
Platt. In: J.A. Smith and W. D. Ross (editors): *The Works of Aristotle.*
Clarendon Press. Oxford. 1958.

7. Aelian (Claudius Aelianus): *On the Characteristics of Animals.*
(In 3 vols.) Translated from the Greek by A.F. Scholfield. Harvard
University Press. Cambridge. 1971-2. See vol. 1, page 145, and vol 2,
page 141.

8. For a compilation of the stories alluding to wind impregnation,
see: Conway Zirkle: Animals impregnated by the wind. *Isis,* Volume 25,
1936. Pages 95-130.

9. Pierre Darmon: *Le Mythe de la Procréation à l'âge Baroque.* J.J.
Pauvert. Paris. 1977. Pages 121-122.

10. Denis Diderot: *Entretien entre D'Alambert et Diderot.* In:
Oeuvres. Gallimard (collection *La Pléiade*), Paris. 1951. Pages 873-885.

11. Peter C. Hoppe and Karl Illmensee: Microsurgically produced
homozygous-diploid uniparental mice. Proceedings of the National
Academy of Sciences of U.S.A. Volume 74, 1977. Pages 5657-5661.

12. James McGrath and Davor Solter: Completion of mouse embryogenesis requires both the maternal and paternal genome. *Cell*, volume 37, 1984. Pages 179-184.

13. Charles Augustin Vandermonde: *Essai sur la Manière de Perfectionner l'Espèce Humaine*. Vincent, Paris. 1756. See chapter 6. Page 392.

14. Nicolas Malebranche: *De la Recherche de la Vérité*. Book 2, part 1. In: *Oeuvres*. (In 2 vols.). Gallimard (collection *Pléiade*) Paris. 1979.

15. *Id.*: Book 2, part 1, chapter 7: pages 178-180.

16. The malformations mentioned appear diagrammed in: J. Edgar Morison: *Foetal and Neonatal Pathology*. Part II, (Adaptation to Extrauterine Existence), chapter 15, entitled "Conditions interfering with normal post-natal development and growth." Butterworths, London. 1963. Page 390.

17. J. A. Blondel: *Sur la Forme de l'Imagination des Femmes Enceintes sur le Foetus*. Gilbert Langerak & Theodor Lucht. Leyden. 1737.

18. D.J. Barker: The fetal origins of adult disease. The Wellcome Foundation Lecture 1994. *Proceedings of the Royal Society*. Volume 262; 1994, pp 37-43. See also a review in: D.J. Barker: Growth in utero and coronary heart disease. *Nutrition Reviews*. Volume 54 (Part 2); 1996 (Feb.), pp S1-7.

19. The following works deal mainly with audition in the fetus, and secondarily with other forms of sense perception: J.P. Lecanuet, C. Granier-Defere, amd M.C. Busnel: Differential autditory reactiveness as a function of stimulus characteristics and state. *Seminars in Perinatology*. Volume 13; 1989, pp 421-429; Kenneth Gerhardt and Robert M. Abrams: Fetal hearing: characterization of the stimulus and response. *Seminars in Perinatology*. Volume 20; 1996, pp 11-20; Denis Querleu, Xavier Renard, Fabienne Versyp, and Laurence Paris-Delrue: Fetal hearing. *European Journal of Obstetrics & Gynecology and Reproductive Biology*. Volume 28; 1988, pp. 191-212.

20. A.W.Liley: The foetus as a personality. *Australian and New Zealand Journal of Psychiatry*. Volume 6; 1972, pp 99-105.

21. Janet L. Hopson: Fearfully and wonderfully made. *Psychology Today*. Volume 31, No. 5; (Oct.) 1998, pp 44-48, 78.

22. T. Humphrey: Some correlations between the appearance of human fetal reflexes and the development of the nervous system. *Progress in Brain Research*. Volume 4; 1964, pp 93-135.

23. R. F. Thompson and W. A. Spencer: Habituation: a model phenomenon for the study of neuronal substrates of behavior. Psychological Review. Volume 73; 1966, pp. 16-43.

24. Richard Lewontin: "Darwin's Revolution." Chapter 2 in: It Ain't Necessarily So. The Dream of the Human Genome and Other Illusions. New York Review Books. New York, 2000.

Before Being Born, You Must Take Sides

1. Aelius Lampridius was one of six authors who wrote the collection known as Scriptores Historiae Augustae. Nothing is known about them. The passage in which the birth of Diadematus is told was transcribed and translated by Nicole Belmont, in her scholarly book, Les Signes de la Naissance. Étude de Représentations Symboliques Associées aux Nasissances Singulières. Plon, Paris. 1971.

2. See The Complete Works of Aristotle. The Revised Oxford Translation. (In two volumes). Vol. 1. Edited by Jonathan Barnes. Princeton, Bollingen Series LXXI-2. 1984. Page 1017.

3. Immanuel Kant: Von dem ersten Grunde des Unterschiedes der Gegenden im Raume. Translated as: "Concerning the ultimate ground of the differentiation of directions in space." In: Theoretical Philosophy, 1755-1770. The Cambridge Edition of the Works of Immanuel Kant. Cambridge University Press. 1992.

4. Roger Caillois: La Dissymétrie. Gallimard, Paris. 1973.

5. For laterality and genetics, see: M. Reiss and G. Reiss: Earedness and handedness: distribution in a German sample with some family data. Cortex, Volume 35 (3): 1999. Pages 403-412; M. Reiss: Genetic associations between lateral signs. Anthropologischer Anzeiger. Volume 57 (1), 1999. Pages 61-68.; M. Annett: Handedness and cerebral dominance: the right shift theory. Journal of Neuropsychiatry and Clinical Neurosciences. Volume 10 (4), 1998. Pages 459-469; M.C. Corballis: The genetics and evolution of handedness. Psychological Review. Volume 104 (4), 1997. Pages 714-727.

6. Pliny the Elder: Natural History. (In ten vols.) Translated by H. Rackham. Loeb Classics. Harvard University Press. Cambridge. 1989. Vol. 2, Page 537.

7. Nicole Belmont. Loc. cit. See note 1.

8. See: "Lie, presentation, attitude and position of the fetus." Chapter 10 in F. Gary Cunningham, Paul C. MacDonald, Kenneth Leveno, and Larry C. Gilstrap, III: William's Obstetrics. 10th edition. Appleton & Lange. New York, 1993.

9. P.J. Danielian, J.Wang, and M.H. Hall: Long term outcome by method of delivery of fetuses in breech presentation at term: population based follow up. *BMJ* (British Medical Journal) Vol. 312; June 1996. Pages 14551-1453. See also several letters of commentary published in *BMJ,*
in reaction to the article by Danielian and collaborators: BMJ Vol. 313, September 1996. Pages 817-818.

10. F. Cardini and H. Weixin: Moxibustion for correction of breech presentation: a randomized control trial. *Journal of the American Medical Association*. Volume 280 (No. 18), November 11, 1998. Pages 1580-1584.

11. Louis Frédéric: *Buddhism*. Flammarion Iconographic Guides. Flammarion, New York, 1995. Page 88.

12. Pliny: *Natural History*. (In 10 vols.). Vol. 2. Translated by H. Rackham. Loeb Classics, Harvard University Press, Cambridge, Mass. Book VII, chapter xvi-72. Page 553.

From Dividual to Individual

1. I used a Spanish translation of the colloquium. See: Desiderio Erasmo Roterdamo: "*El filósofo y la parida*." In: *Obras Escogidas*. Translated from the Latin by Lorenzo Riber. Aguilar, Madrid. 1956. Pages 1134-1148.

2. Albert Jacquard: *Pour Une Terre de 10 Milliards d'Hommes*. Zulma, Toulouse. 1998.

3. For discussion of the establishment of the embryo's body plan, see: John Kimble: An ancient molecular mechanism for establishing embryonic polarity. *Science*. Vol. 266 (October 28); 1994. Pages 577-578; Theories of biological pattern formation. *Philosophical Transactions of the Royal Society of London (Biology)* Vol. 295; 1981. Pages 425-617; Wolpert L.: Pattern formation in biological development. *Scientific American*. Vol. 239 (Number 4); 1978. Pages 154-164.

4. José de Cadalso: *Cartas Marruecas*. Espasa-Calpe. Madrid. 1975. Page 55.

5. Dorothy Nelkin and M. Susan Lindee: *The DNA Mystique. The Gene As a Cultural Icon*. W.H. Freeman and Co., New York. 1995. Page 8.

6. François Jacob: *La Souris, La Mouche et L'Homme*. Odile Jacob. Paris. 2000.

7. See: Paul Hillyard: *The Book of the Spider*. Random House, New York. 1994. The biotechnology company pursuing the industrial

recovery of spider silk by insertion of the pertinent gene into goat's mammatry glands is *Nexia*, whose Web site is *<nexiabiotech.com>*. See also: Tirrell DA: Putting a new spin on spider silk. *Science*: volume 271; 1996. Pages 139-40.

8. A. Colman: Production of proteins in the milk of transgenic livestock: Problems, solutions and successes. *American Journal of Clinical Nutrition*. Volume 63, 1996. Pages 639S-645S.

9. L.M. Houdebine: Production of pharmaceutical proteins from transgenic animals. *Journal of Biotechnology*. Vol. 14, 1994. Pages 269-287.

10. Peter Singer: *Practical Ethics*, 2nd edition. Cambridge University Press. 1999.

11. Florence Burgat: *Les habits de la cruauté*. In: Boris Cyrulknik (editor): *Si Les Lions Pouvaient Parler*. Gallimard, Paris. 1998. Pages 1220-1243.

Crossing the Valley of the Shadow of Birth

1. Walter Burkert: Ancient Mystery Cults. Harvard University Press, Cambridge. 1987. P.89.

2. Fernand Lamaze: *Painless Childbirth: Psychoprophylactic Method*. Regnery, Chicago. 1970.

3. As an example of medical litterature supportive of Lamaze's method, see: Hughey M.J., Mc Elin T.W., and Young T.: Outcome of Lamaze-prepared patients. *Obstetrics & Gynecology*, Vol. 51, 1978. Pages 643 & ff.

4. Birth related customs and folklore are quoted from G.J. Engelmann's book, that appeared in German language edition as: *Die Geburt bei den Urvolkern. Eine Darstellung der Entwicklung der heuitigen Geburstkunde aus dem natürlichen und unbewussten Gebrauche aller Rassen*. Vienna, 1884. This work exists in English as *Labor Among Primitive Peoples*. St Louis, J.H. Chambers. 1882.

5. The relation between witches and midwifery is extensively dealt with in: Thomas Rogers Forbes: The Midwife and the Withch. Yale University Press, New Haven. 1960. See also: J.H. Aveling: *English Midwives*. London, AMS Press. 1977.

6. Nancy Mitford: *The Sun King*. Penguin Books, New York. 1966.

7. Ralph Jackson: *Doctors and Diseases in the Roman Empire*. British Museum Press, London. 1988. Page 86.

8. For a fine biography of Madame du Coudray, see: Nina Rattner

Gelbart : *The King's Midwife. A History and Mistery of Madame Du Coudray.* University of California Press. Berkeley. 1998.

9. The article on parturition is under the letter "A", (*Accouchement, Accoucheuse*), volume one of Denis Diderot: *Encyclopédie.* Critical and annotated edition presented by John Lough and Jacques Proust. Hermann, Paris. 1976. Pages 237-242.

10. Dorothy C. Wertz: What birth has done for doctors. *Women & Health.* Vol. 8, 1983. Pages 7-24.

11. Julien Joseph Virey: *De l'Influence des Femmes Sur le Goût Dans la Littérature et les Beaux Arts Pendant le XVIIe et XVIIIe Siècles.* Paris. 1810. Page 68.

12. Charles François de Menville, Dr.: *Histoire Médicale et Philosophique de la Femme.* Paris. 1845. Page 79

13. Philippe Hecquet: *De l'Indécence aux Hommes à Accoucher les Femmes, et de l'Obligation des Femmes à Nourrir Leurs Enfants.* J. Etienne. Paris. 1708.

14. Nicolas Venette: *La Génération de l'Homme, ou Tableau de l'Amour Conjugal Considéré dans l'Etat du Mariage.* Parme, 1696 (first published in 1685). For a study of this enormously popular work, which was reprinted many times, see: Roy Porter: Spreading carnal knowledge or selling dirt cheap? Nicolas Venette's *Tableau de l'Amour Conjugal* in 18th century England. *Journal of European Studies.* Vol. 14, 1984. Pages 233-255.

15. Quoted in: J.W. Leavitt: Science enters the birthing room: obstetrics in America since the eighteenth century. *Journal of American History.* Vol. 70; 1983. Pages 282-286.

16. R.A. Sosa and J.M. Cupoli: The birthing process: effect on the parents. *Clinics in Perinatology.* Vol. 8, number 1, 1981. Page 197.

17. A.P. Clark: The influence of position of the patient in labor in causing uterine inertia and pelvic disturbances. *Journal of the American Medical Association* Vol. 16; 1891. Page 431.

18. Quoted by Yvonne Barlow, in: Childbirth: management of labor through the ages. *Nursing Times* Vol. 90. Number 35 (Aug. 31), 1994. Pages 41-43.

19. The 1200-page work, considered to be the most authoritative texbook of the specialty in the early part of the twentieth century, is Joseph B. De Lee's *Principles and Practice of Obstetrics* , W.B. Saunders. St. Louis, Mo., first printed in 1913, and then reprinted many times until 1940.

20. Richard W. Wertz and Dorothy Wertz: *Lying-in. A History of Childirth in America.* Yale University Press. New Haven. 1989.

21. Jessica Mitford: *The American Way of Birth*. Dutton. New York. 1992.

22. Some of the mentioned criticisms are reviewed in the following bibliography, which does not attempt to be complete. J. W. Leavitt: *Brought to Bed: Childbearing in America: 175 0-1950*. Oxford University Press. Oxford. 1986; A. Oakley: *The Captured Womb: A History of the Medical Care of Pregnant Women*. Basil Blackwell. Oxford. 1984; M. Sandelowski: *Pain, Pleasure, and American Childbirth: From the Twilight Sleep to the Read Method*. 1914-1960. Greenwood Press, London. 1984; S. Arms: *Immaculate Deception: A New Look at Women and Childbirth in America*. Houghton Mifflin. Boston. 1975.

23. See, for a development of this thesis, Donald Caton, M.D.: *What a Blessing She Had Chloroform. The Medical and Social Response to the Pain of Childbirth From 1800 to the Present*. Yale University Press. New Haven. 1999.

24. Interview quoted in: Robbie E. Davis-Floyd: *Birth as an American Rite of Passage*. University of California Press. Berkeley. 1992. Page 55.

25. Mary Field: The jewel in the crown. Clitoral massage as an analgesia for labor. *Chilbirth Alternatives Quarterly*. Vol.6., Num.4; winter 1984-1985. Pages 4-5.

26. Alexandre Minkowski: *L'Art de Naître*. Odile Jacob, Paris. 1987. Page 220.

The Flowers of Evil in the Garden of Biology

1. Arthur Schopenhauer: *The World as Will and Representation*. Translated from the German by E.J.F. Payne. In two vols. Dover. New York. 1966. Vol. 2, page 467.

2. Quoted by Erasmus of Rotterdam, in *Adages* (*Op. cit.*).

3. Herodotus: *The Histories*. Translated by Aubrey de Sélincourt. Penguin. New York. 1972. Book 5. Page 342.

4. W. K. C. Guthrie: *A History of Greek Philosophy*. (In two vols). Cambridge University Press, Cambridge. 1966 (reprinted 1980). Vol. Two. Page 47.

5. Jean Rostand: *L'Aventure Avant la Naissance (Du Germe au Nouveau-Né)*. Gonthier. Paris. 1953. Page 60.

6. Quoted by Nicole Le Douarin in her book, *Des Chimères, Des Clones et Des Gènes*. Odile Jacob. Paris 2000. Pages 115-116.

7. E. Mayr: *The Growth of Biological Thought*. Belknap Press (Harvard). Cambridge. 1982. Page 473.

8. Stephen Jay Gould: *Ontogeny and Philogeny*. Belknap Press (Harvard) Cambridge. 1977.

9. Guillaume Mauquest de la Motte: *Traité complet des accouchements naturels, non naturels et contre nature, expliqué dans un grand nombre d'observations et de réflections sur l'art d'accoucher*. D'Houry. Paris. 1722.

10. Joseph Antoine Toussaint Cangiamila: *Abrégé del'embryologie sacrée, ou traité des devoirs des prêtres, des médecins, des chirurgiens et des sages femmes envers les enfans qui sont dans le sein de leur mère, traduit de l'italien par l'Abbé Dinouart*. (Site and publisher not stated). 1775. This is a French translation from the 1745 Italian edition.

11. Mircea Eliade: *The Sacred and the Profane. The Nature of Religion*. Translated from the French by Willard R. Trask. Harper and Row. New York, 1961. See especially chapter three, entitled "The Sacredness of Nature and Cosmic Religion." Pages 116-159.

12. Kenneth Luehrsen and Virginia Walbot: Firefly luciferase as a reporter for plant gene expression studies. *Promega Notes Magazine*. No. 44, 1991. Page 24. See also: Emily Reiter: Glowing plants indicate internal clocks in action. *Alaska Science Forum* (University of Alaska Fairbanks publication). Article 1264, Dec. 8, 1995.

13. Abigail Trafford: Octuplets and other babies. *Washington Post*, January 12, 1999.

14. Reported in 20/20 ABC News March 31, 1999.

15. To read the interview, see internet address <http://abcnews.go .com/onair/2020transcripts>.

16. Lori B. Andrews: *The Clone Age. Adventures in the New World of Reproductive Technology*. Henry Holt. New York, 1999. With an afterword in 2000.

17. *Id.*, page 37.

List of Illustrations

p. 36, 110: W. Blair Bell: *The Principles of Gynaecology.* 3rd ed. London. Baillère, Tindall & Cox. 1919.

p. 57: Edward Casp. Jac. von Siebold: *Abbildungen aus dem Gesammtgebiete der teoretisch-praktischen Geburtshülfe nebst beschreibender Erklärung.* Reutlingen. Jakob Noa Ensslin. 1836. Reprinted from the Berlin 1829 edition.

p. 94: J. Edgar Morison: *Foetal and Neonatal Pathology.* 2nd. Edition, London. Butterworths 1963. (Fig. 105 on page 390: "Anencephaly & Iniencephaly").

p. 96: Isidore Geoffroy Saint-Hilaire: *Histoire Générale et Particulière de l'Organisation chez l'Homme et les Animaux.* (In 3 Vols.). Brussels. Hauman, Cattoir et Cie. 1837.

p. 117: Francis H. Ramsbotham: *Principles and Practice of Obsteric Medicine.* Philadelphia. Lea & Blanchard. 1847.

p. 183: Ernst Haeckel: *The History of Creation, or the Development of the Earth and its Inhabitants, by the Action of Natural Causes.* (In 2 vols.) Vol. 1. Translated by E. Ray Lankester. London. Henry S. King & Co., 1876.